Chronicling the Tuskegee Syphilis Study

Essays, Research Writings, Commentaries,
and Other Documented Works

Obiora N. Anekwe, Ed.D
and
Ejinkonye C. Anekwe, Ph.D

ISBN: 1492837202
ISBN 13: 9781492837206

About the Cover Art:

The art collage, *Human Subjects*, by Obiora N. Anekwe, shows seven African-American men who participated in the Tuskegee Syphilis Study. The faces of the men are blackened to protect their identities and to represent the concept of being invisible human subjects, or guinea pigs, experimented upon by public health practitioners. There are black shadows behind each man, representing the wide effect this unethical study had on many black men who do not trust the Public Health Service and, therefore, have not participated in future Public Health Service clinical trials.

The artwork also illustrates how African-American male participants involved in the Tuskegee Syphilis Study were depicted-with their shirts off and faces shown-in the photographs made by the study to document the disease. As the artist, I abstractly blackened the faces of the men to further emphasize their physical attributes such as bodily strength, which helped to promote the unfounded medical stereotype that the African-American male body was more physically resistant to syphilis than the bodies of men of other ethnicities.

Obiora N. Anekwe
December 11, 2012
Brooklyn, New York

16 by 20 inches
Canvas paper, gouache paint, soft pastels, black and white charcoal pencils, and copy paper

Original images provided by the National Archives and Records Administration, Southeast Region, Morrow, Georgia.

About the Authors:

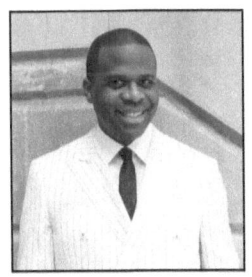

Photographer: Brittany Okpagu

Obiora N. Anekwe was born in Alabama on the campus of Tuskegee Institute (now Tuskegee University) in the John A. Andrew Memorial Hospital. Reared in Lagos, Nigeria, he attended the University of Lagos Staff School as a child. He is a graduate of Clark Atlanta University (BA, mass media arts), Tuskegee University (MEd, counseling and student development), and Auburn University (EdD, educational leadership). His early educational experiences influenced his commitment to learning, presenting, and conducting research in international education in Germany, Italy, Poland, and Scotland. Obiora is currently pursuing a Master of Science in Bioethics at Columbia University in New York City. Before coming to Columbia, he worked as a counselor, instructor, and educational coordinator at Tuskegee University. In addition, he has taught as an adjunct instructor in Educational Foundations at Auburn University.

As an emerging educational bioethicist, Obiora has received additional training in bioethics, health care, and clinical ethics from the Kennedy Institute of Ethics at Georgetown University, Union Graduate College, and Mount Sinai School of Medicine. He is a member of the American Society for Bioethics and Humanities and the New York Academy of Sciences. He has published in the field of education.

His first book, *Celebrating Life at 24 Hampton Place*, chronicles the Igbo traditional life and home-going celebrations of his great-aunt, Mrs. Catherine N. Anekwe.

Dr. Obiora N. Anekwe resides in Brooklyn, New York, with his wife, Rev. Alexis Southerland Anekwe.

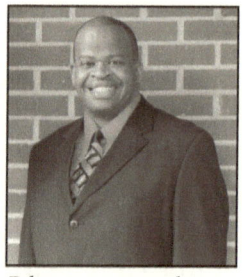

Ejinkonye Anekwe was born on August 9, 1972 at John Andrew Hospital on the campus of Tuskegee Institute (now Tuskegee University). His mother, Emma Anekwe, is a retired educator and a former medical technologist at Tuskegee University. His father, Gregory Anekwe, is a retired biochemistry professor who also taught at Tuskegee University as an associate professor of biochemistry. In 1975, at the age of three, Ejinkonye, his brother, Obiora, and his parents moved to Lagos, Nigeria. There he was exposed to Nigerian culture and attended elementary school at the University of Lagos Staff School. In 1981, Ejinkonye returned to the United States with his brother and mother at the age of nine. Ejinkonye and his brother grew up in Columbus, Georgia, where they were raised by their mother and maternal grandparents, SFC (Ret.) Arthur A. Maddox and Eliza W. Maddox, a retired principal. Ejinkonye finished Carver High School in 1990, graduating seventh out of a senior class of 138 students.

After graduating high school, Ejinkonye attended Clark Atlanta University on a scholarship sponsored by the United States Federal Government. In 1994, he graduated with a BS in biology, also graduating with distinction from the University's honors program. In 1996, Ejinkonye was awarded a fellowship to study cytogenetics at Tuskegee University, where he conducted research on amphibian chromosomes. His thesis, "Comparative Cytogenetic Analyses of *Rana pipiens* Normal Tissue Derived Cell Lines, RpKID and RpLIV," attempted to ascertain the potential of the analyzed cell lines as suitable *in vitro* controls for a tumor-derived, *Rana pipiens* cell line called PNKT-4B, or Pronephric Kidney Tumor Series B. The line was derived from the Luckè tumor, which is a pronephric tumor found in *Rana pipiens* tadpoles. In 1999, he graduated with an MS degree in biology from Tuskegee University.

From 2001 to 2002, Ejinkonye worked on his master's degree in public administration at Columbus State University in Georgia. His master's thesis, "Survey Attitudes toward Stem Cell Research," dealt with public attitudes regarding stem cell research policies. In 2002, Ejinkonye graduated with an MPA degree in general government.

In 2004, Ejinkonye began doctoral classes in the Department of Conflict Analysis and Resolution in the Graduate School of Humanities and Social Sciences at Nova Southeastern University. His dissertation was titled "The Effects of Age, Ethnicity, Gender, and Socioeconomic Background on Responses to Conflict among Community College Students." In 2012, he graduated with a PhD in humanities and social sciences, specializing in conflict analysis and resolution.

Ejinkonye is currently an adjunct instructor in biology at Chattahoochee Valley Community College in Phenix City, Alabama. He has worked as a biology instructor at Columbus Technical College in Georgia. He has also worked as a science and math tutor.

Chronicling the Tuskegee Syphilis Study:
Essays, Research Writings, Commentaries,
and Other Documented Works

Obiora N. Anekwe, Ed.D
and
Ejinkonye C. Anekwe, Ph.D

TABLE OF CONTENTS

FOREWORD

In 1997, unbeknown to me, I began the journey of understanding the Tuskegee Syphilis Study. Although learning more about the study interested me, I did not realize that it would encompass so much of my life. For me, this journey began when, as a graduate student, I watched the nationally televised apology ceremony by US President Bill Clinton. One decade later, I am even more passionate about telling the story of the men who suffered because of medical neglect.

To my surprise, due to the amount of commentaries, essays, papers and other forms of written text about the Tuskegee Syphilis Study over the years, I had a great deal of the book completed by the end of 2012. In 2013, I enlisted my brother's expertise and asked him to cowrite the book with me because of our shared interest in bioethics and the Tuskegee Syphilis Study. Since my brother and I were both born in the hospital where the syphilis study took place, and since we're both graduates of Tuskegee University, I found it highly appropriate that we write a book about such as significant topic in North American history.

Because our book is a compilation of various writings during different periods of our research about the Tuskegee Syphilis Study, some themes or topics within some essays may seem repetitious, but each individual section of the book has a point to make. This form of repetition also serves as a means to highlight particular themes or topics that may need greater emphasis. Some essays and reports in chapter three were written in response to assigned readings, to which the reader will see occasional references. Our primary goal was to compile a body of work from essays to papers about the Tuskegee Syphilis Study in order to provide the reader with a framework for further discussion. My brother and I are both pleased that you have decided to join us on this fascinating journey.

~ Obiora N. Anekwe

CHAPTER 1:
DEFINING BIOETHICS

Most people are unaware of the meaning of the word *bioethics* and its real life implications in our day-to-day existence. Bioethics can be defined as the study of the ethics (the rightness or wrongness of an action) in medicine, health care, and related fields. But it can also be defined in broader terms, which gives the field greater depth.

Historically, the term *bioethics* is rooted in the field of medical ethics. Bioethics has been affiliated with such areas as biomedical sciences and biotechnology. It can also be described as the study of ethics in the life (bio) sciences. For our discussions here, in relation to the Tuskegee Syphilis Study, bioethics can include the study of the moral, historical, ethical, philosophical, humanistic, and justice facets of health care and medical practice.

But the definition of bioethics itself can be more broad and flexible. It can study, research, and critically analyze scientific themes through artistic, philosophical, and legalistic interpretations in order to translate broad and specific meanings. Even the definitions laid out before the reader do not give sufficient justice to the full extent of bioethics. Due to its emergence within the last forty years, many new challenges in human existence will redefine the ethical applicability of the sciences in the twenty-first century.

CHAPTER 2

RESEARCH HISTORY OF SCHOLARS

Rooted in Tuskegee: My Personal Journey to Tell the Story

Obiora N. Anekwe
February, 2013

How did my journey toward documenting the Tuskegee Syphilis Study begin? Why am I so passionate about this issue? And why did I choose to tell this story? These are just a few questions that I hope to answer in this essay. For me, it all began at my birth on September 10, 1974 at the John A. Andrew Memorial Hospital in Tuskegee Institute, Alabama. The hospital was the site of the Tuskegee Syphilis Study, which concluded two years before my birth. My mother, Emma Jeanette Anekwe (Maddox), was a medical technologist at the hospital during the time period of the syphilis study. My father, Gregory E. Anekwe, PhD, was an associate professor of biochemistry at Tuskegee University and researcher at the George Washington Carver Research Foundation.

When I was ten months old, in 1975, my family and I moved to Lagos, Nigeria, where my father worked at the University of Lagos as chair of the Department of Biochemistry in the College of Medicine. As a child growing up in Lagos, I was exposed to the visual arts that influenced me to study art, oral history, and science. These three particular areas fueled my passion to eventually examine the Tuskegee Syphilis Study through my formal education and through my personal experience of working as a counselor and professor at Tuskegee University.

When my family and I returned to the United States in 1981, when I was six, I knew very little about the Tuskegee Syphilis Study. The general public became exposed to the study itself in 1972, two years before my own birth. At an early age, I spoke the Yoruba language and broken English. Eventually, through a speech therapist, I learned standard English. But as a result, I developed a stutter, which affected me for years and became a great challenge. Once I overcame this challenge, I began to focus on how I could tell the stories of other people who struggled through their own challenges. As a graduate student studying counseling at Tuskegee University, I was exposed to details of the Tuskegee Syphilis Study through the nationally televised public apology presented from the White House in 1997. President Clinton gave the apology on behalf of the federal government because of its sponsorship of the study. As I remember, the apology seemed to be of monumental importance to the victims who attended the event at the White House. For me, though I didn't realize it at the time, studying this event in US history would become one of my life's passions.

After I completed my master's degree at Tuskegee University in 1999, I began work on my doctorate in educational leadership at Auburn University. During this period, the National Center for Bioethics in Research and Health Care at Tuskegee University was in its primary stages of development. As I studied more about educational ethics, law, educational policy, and curriculum development, I began to integrate many of my coursework themes into the study of bioethics due to its strong emphasis in ethics and philosophy. Since my senior year in high school, when I took my first philosophy course in political philosophy, ethics and philosophy have always interested me. Therefore, merging my interest in these areas, in addition to my developing interest in the Tuskegee Syphilis Study, seemed a natural springboard to obtaining a master's degree in bioethics. After my doctoral studies, I took a summer intensive certificate training course during the summer of 2009 at the Kennedy Institute of Ethics at Georgetown University in Washington, DC. I studied under the tutelage of Edmund D. Pellegrino, MD, one of the premier scholars in the field of bioethics. After this course, I decided that I wanted to formally explore my interest in the Tuskegee Syphilis Study by applying to a hybrid online and on-site bioethics master's program at Union Graduate College in Schenectady, New York. I was accepted into the program during the summer of 2010 and began my journey to learn more about this significant study.

After a year and a half of taking courses at Union, I decided that I wanted to study directly at the center of the bioethics community in New York. In the summer of 2012, I moved to Brooklyn, New York, where I lived in the home of my great-aunt, Catherine N. Anekwe, with the hopes of transferring to Columbia University in New York City in order to complete my master's degree in bioethics. During that summer, I was accepted into the program, and I began a series of art collages based on the Tuskegee Syphilis Study, which serve as a means to create a sense of visual healing for victims of the study and to tell their story in a more visual manner.

The path to telling the story of the victims and their families has been a tremendous learning experience beginning in 2010 with my video interview with Elizabeth Sims (deceased), founder of the Shiloh Community Restoration Foundation and family member to renowned victims of the syphilis study.

Ever since my first encounter with Mrs. Sims, I was determined to try to find as many ways to tell the story of these brave warriors, who are known to be the research participants of one of the longest government-sponsored clinical trials in US history (1932–1972).

It has been an honor and privilege to give a voice and a face to a story that can never be forgotten.

My Experiences with Research and Bioethics
Ejinkonye C. Anekwe
February, 2013

I was literally born into a scientific setting on August 9, 1972, at John A. Andrew Hospital on the campus of a world-renowned institution, Tuskegee Institute (now Tuskegee University). My parents are Dr. Gregory E. Anekwe, a retired biochemistry professor and researcher, and Emma Anekwe, a former medical technologist and retired educator. Almost two years later, my brother, Dr. Obiora Anekwe, was born at the same hospital on September 10, 1974. The hospital, as I learned through my experiences at Tuskegee University, was the site of unethical experiments conducted at the school under the infamous Tuskegee Syphilis Study.

My first foray into science came at a young age when my father took me to his job as a professor in the Department of Chemistry at the College of Medicine, University of Lagos, in Lagos, Nigeria. I did not understand what chemistry sets were at five years old, but I was fascinated by them. As I got older, I started reading science books in the elementary school library at Carver Elementary School in Columbus, GA. My first summer program in science was in 1987 at Columbus College (now Columbus State University). It was called Science Challenge. I used to assist fellow high school students and professors in collecting water samples from local creeks and testing them for water quality. The experience was one of many more to come.

In 1990, I was awarded a scholarship—the Research Careers for Minorities in the Geosciences (RCMS)—to attend Clark Atlanta

University. Through the scholarship, I participated in internships at Emory University in Atlanta, GA, Pontifica Universidad Catòlica Madre y Maestra (Mother and Teacher Pontifical Catholic University) in Santiago, Dominican Republic, and the Northwest Fisheries Science Center in Seattle, WA. At Emory, I participated in a project known as the Reforestation Project. I helped by writing background data on global warming. In the Dominican Republic, I participated in an effort by the country to reduce deforestation through sustainable development of natural resources such as forests, fish farms, and high-altitude farms. At Northwest Fisheries Science Center, I learned how to catch English Sole and extract its stomach contents so that the research team could use those samples as evidence in the *Exxon Valdez* trial. I worked at Northwest Fisheries after graduating from Clark Atlanta in June 1994.

I had experiences in environmental science and wanted to pursue a master's degree two years after graduation. I entered the biology department at Tuskegee University as a graduate student. As part of my master's degree requirement, I analyzed chromosomes taken from normal-derived *Rana pipiens* (northern leopard frog) liver and kidney cell lines. The research from these cell lines was used to make a comparison to a tumor-derived *Rana pipiens* cell line, PNKT-4B. The goal of the study was to ascertain the effectiveness of the normal-derived cell line as a suitable control group against the tumor-derived cell line. The name of my master's thesis was "Comparative Cytogenetic Analyses of *Rana pipiens* Normal Tissue Derived Cell Lines, RpKID and RpLIV."

In addition to my research with amphibian cells, I was introduced to HeLa cells, cervical cancer cells extracted from Henrietta Lacks, an African-American woman who was afflicted with an aggressive form of the disease. After she died, her cervix was removed from her body, and her cancerous cells were harvested in bioreactors throughout the United States. It just so happened that the same HeLa cells that I was using as practice for my eventual research were made at the Carver Research Foundation at Tuskegee University. At the time when I was a graduate student, I was unaware of the fact that these HeLa cells were taken without the knowledge of the Lacks family. Tuskegee University was known as a HeLa cell factory because the George Washington Carver Research Foundation operated a bioreactor that grew millions of these cancer cells. In fact, Tuskegee University had the largest collection of HeLa cells in the world. The school used to export the cells to research centers throughout the world. Tuskegee University's biology department had so many HeLa cells that we practiced using them for chromosomal analyses such as G-banding, C-banding, and AgNOR-banding. It was amazing how many cells graduate students and research scientists used in the course of their studies over the past half-century.

When I graduated with a master of science degree in biology from Tuskegee University in 1999, I wanted to migrate out of laboratory research and to integrate natural sciences with social issues. In order to accomplish this, I needed to gain some experience in sociology. In 2001, I enrolled in the public administration program at Columbus State University. There I learned about the functions of the United States government. Since I was trained in biology, I decided to write my master's thesis on stem cell research. More specifically, I wanted to discover the attitudes of randomly selected individuals toward embryonic stem cell research. I was anticipating that religion and educational level would have a bearing on support of stem cell research. I based this assumption on previous research that suggested that some religious groups opposed embryonic cloning. The thesis, titled "Survey Attitudes toward Stem Cell Research," sampled 113 respondents from the Columbus, GA metropolitan area. The results indicated that most respondents opposed embryonic stem cell research, regardless of education and religion. I stated in my research that the results may have been due to a lack of understanding of embryonic stem cells. That may very well be the case, but in my opinion, many people may be wary of controversial human research. This is understandable given the horrors of the Tuskegee Syphilis Study. As I examined the ramifications of stem cell research, I pondered the potential for abuse. For instance, I mentioned that several countries, such as Germany and the United States enacted laws that banned federal funding for embryonic cloning, in part to prevent medical abuse. After several years of such a ban, the administration of President Barrack Obama reversed the ban, thus allowing federal funding for embryonic stem cell research. Now, instead of eugenic aspirations, many researchers are interested in curing diseases among the sick and elderly.

In August 2002, I graduated from Columbus State University with a master's degree in public administration. Shortly thereafter, I wished to continue exploring the social aspects of scientific research. However, I wanted to concentrate on studying how groups of people respond to stressful situations such as conflicts. In hindsight, the exploration into human behavior would come in handy with understanding healing strategies used for family members of the victims of the Tuskegee Syphilis Study. In 2003, I applied to the Conflict Resolution program in the Graduate School of Humanities and Social Sciences at Nova Southeastern University (Fort Lauderdale, FL). I was accepted into the program that year, but I postponed enrollment until 2004 so that I might better understand the field of conflict resolution. By January 2004, I took my first classes in conflict analysis and resolution.

I concentrated my research on conflict resolution among community college students. My dissertation was titled, "The Effects of Age, Ethnicity, Gender, and Socioeconomic Background on Conflicts among Community College Students." I sought to understand whether individual student responses to conflicts were based on their social backgrounds. I found that, of the social backgrounds of age, ethnicity, gender, and socioeconomics, the key differences in how community college students responded to conflict were in the social factor of gender. Having earned my PhD in humanities and social sciences in 2012, I intend to perform future research on social factors and conflict, but I would also like to relate the field of conflict resolution to the use of holistic healing of families affected by the Tuskegee Syphilis Study.

Conflict resolution plays a pivotal role in the Tuskegee Syphilis Study. For one thing, the study itself conflicted with the personal autonomy of each individual participant. According to Maslow's hierarchy of needs, autonomy is one of the critical requirements for a human being to survive. Without autonomy, a person has no sense of self. The removal of autonomy by the doctors and scientists at Tuskegee prevented the subjects from experiencing life at its fullest. Thus, conflicts arose between the participants and the researchers who were in charge of the study. Regardless of education level and socioeconomic status, the participants of the Tuskegee Syphilis Study were deprived of the chance to enjoy their lives, and even to be sharecroppers. Instead, their bodies were subjected to pain and torment. To me, this is the ultimate, most personal form of conflict.

I wish to contribute to the understanding of the Tuskegee Syphilis Study by developing holistic healing strategies. These strategies form a part of conflict resolution by examining grievances and pain in the hopes of transforming sadness into hope. One healing strategy that I would like to implement is poetry writing, particularly slam poetry and hip hop. Artists can study the history of the Tuskegee Syphilis Study through interviewing the descendants of the participants. The songs they create can be recorded and sold through an artist-generated website, with the profits going to the family members of the study participants. Advertisements can be placed on YouTube to garner attention and support. This way, young people can understand the history of human experimentation and scientific racism.

CHAPTER 3

BIOETHICAL WRITINGS AND ESSAYS

Obiora N. Anekwe
Essay 1

In my reading of the book *Subjected to Science: Human Experimentation in America before the Second World War* (1995), by Susan E. Lederer, I asked myself whether experiments on animal research subjects is ethical in any form? Professor Peter Singer of Princeton University would surely argue that not only are experimentations on animals unnecessary, but they are unethical due to the universal element and nature of suffering, which all beings share. The interesting aspect for me, in terms of human and animal experimentation, is in suffering that cannot be scientifically measured. Suffering is suffering, and how can anyone measure it scientifically? Another aspect that ties together human and animal experimentation in the 1800s and early 1900s is the lack of informed consent by research subjects. An animal, of course, cannot communicate nor fully comprehend the context of experimentation on the body. Many human beings, such as orphans and the mentally ill, were also not informed of the extent to which experimentation on their bodies could cause irreversible harm. Many such patients suffered lasting wounds and scars from clinical experimentations that supposedly advanced medicine.

I found parallels in this particular article with German and French doctors' disassociation with suffering in the human body. In my observation, their medical attitudes toward extreme human experimentation in the 1800s and early 1900s seem to be a precursor to the unthinkable human experimentations that occurred during World War II under the supervision of Nazi doctors and scientific researchers in concentration camps. The concept of *benevolent deception*, practiced by many medical doctors years before, was later transformed into blatantly deceptive medical practices that influenced such clinical studies as the Tuskegee Syphilis Study (1932–1972) and the Guatemalan Syphilis Study in the 1940s. This sense of *medical disassociation*, which views those who are experimented upon as *the other*, was also highlighted in the article, "An Introduction to the Study of Experimental Medicine," by Claude Bernard. In the latter portion of the article, human suffering is discussed in terms of experimentation, but a common link between the articles by Lederer and Bernard is the notion that human and animal suffering in experimentation was essentially an afterthought for most clinical researchers during the 1800s and early to mid 1900s.

Obiora N. Anekwe
Essay 2

During the summer of 2006, I had the distinct opportunity to visit the Auschwitz-Birkenau Concentration Camp in Krakow, Poland. It was, to say the least, the most real and moving site I have ever experienced. Further, it was shocking to discover to what extent Nazi medical doctors would conduct extreme experimentations on human beings without any recourse for their senseless actions. I was reminded that all humans are capable of the greatest human good and also capable of performing the greatest human evil. The Nuremberg Code was a direct outcome of the unethical medical acts of Nazi doctors who experimented on Jewish and other religious and/or ethnic populations considered unfit to be human. Medical and nonmedical experiments by Nazi doctors correlated with what is often described in bioethics as *bad eugenics*. These doctors wanted to scientifically prove that ethnic populations such as Polish and German Jews were physically and mentally inferior to the ideal race, the Aryan master race. As a result, these doctors did whatever they deemed necessary to prove their beliefs, even to the extent of conducting experiments that ultimately caused the deaths of thousands upon thousands of Jewish people.

I discovered it quite ironic that the Nazi doctors' experimentations and the Tuskegee Syphilis Study are being covered in the readings during a period when I am developing an additional series of art collages correlating the ethical and moral layers of both unethical experiments in world history. My most recent art collage, *Shiloh-Auschwitz,* photographically renders the Shiloh Missionary Baptist Church (where many African-American males were recruited to participate in the Tuskegee Syphilis Study) with an original structure of a watchtower from the Auschwitz Concentration Camp. My reasoning for depicting such a scene was to allow the viewer to see how farm-like and docile communities in both Poland and Alabama were ideal locations for conducting their respective experiments. After completing this art piece and further reflecting upon the book, *The Nazi Doctors and the Nuremberg Code* (1992), edited by George J. Annas and Michael A. Grodin, I concluded that these two comparable experiments, in particular those conducted by Nazi doctors on humankind, are symbolic of our greatest conditional extremes.

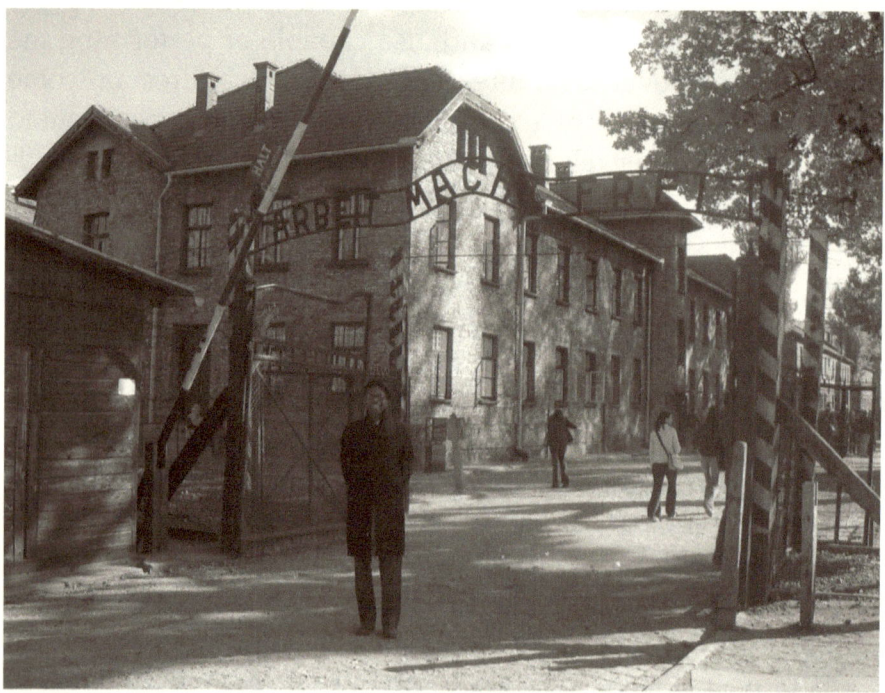

Photograph at the entrance gates of the Auschwitz-Birkenau Concentration Camp in Krakow, Poland

Obiora N. Anekwe
Essay 3

I was born in 1974 on the campus of Tuskegee Institute (now Tuskegee University) in the same hospital where the infamous Tuskegee Syphilis Study occurred. As a young boy who grew up in Lagos, Nigeria, having moved there a year after my birth in the John A. Andrew Memorial Hospital, Tuskegee's role as an institution of higher education and as a small rural town was always portrayed to me as historic in nature. I was unaware of the deeper landscapes of the Tuskegee community and its educational institution until I made various yearly visits with my family to Tuskegee and years later as a graduate student, staff, and faculty member at Tuskegee University. As I grew older, I also grew in my desire to know more about the study that once took place in the hospital I was born in.

In reading the three articles, what struck me the most was the common theme of black identity in each. For me, there was a common theme in how African-American males were viewed by the medical profession of both black and white races, how Nurse Eunice Rivers viewed herself as a medical professional, black women, and moral compass, and how African-Americans viewed themselves—in particular, how black medical professionals and administrators viewed the African-American male participants in the study based on socioeconomic or even educational differences. It seemed as if the men experimented upon were viewed as invisible men, to borrow a concept from author Ralph Ellison, with little to no regard for their life histories, their medical pain and agony, or even their informed consent. In Susan M. Reverby's detailed book reading, *Examining Tuskegee: The Infamous Syphilis Study and Its Legacy*, it was of particular interest to me to understand how the role of silence and secrecy dominated the perpetuation of the syphilis study for forty years. In reading *Tuskegee's*

Truths: Rethinking the Tuskegee Syphilis Study, by Susan M Reverby, I was struck by the letters between and among the Public Health Service doctors, the Tuskegee Institute administration, and officials in the Macon County Health Department. These letters serve as a means to understand why Macon County, Alabama, was selected for the syphilis study, while bringing insight into the misguided medical perceptions of the African-American male body and its physical reaction to syphilis. But most significantly, all three articles demonstrate that the Tuskegee Syphilis Study was a real case study of *what not to do* in human experimentation.

Obiora N. Anekwe
Essay 4

The three articles highlighted in this essay seemed to have one thematic connection: a universal or federally mandated compensation system for children adversely affected by vaccinations. First, the Colgrove and Murray articles centered especially on a federally mandated system of compensation for such victims through the National Vaccine Injury Compensation Program, which was a result of the National Childhood Vaccine Injury Act of 1986. As I read through the various court cases that eventually led to the federally mandated program, I thought about how the program helps a vulnerable population that cannot advocate for itself, other than through parental involvement and initiative. Then I also wondered if other vulnerable populations that were victims of unethical clinical trials could also have a federally mandated compensation system initiated from a federal act. To me, it would seem logical, since many people who were participants in such studies at Willowbrook and Tuskegee were also vulnerable participants who were clearly uninformed and negatively affected by participating in unethical clinical trials.

The articles by Colgrove and Murray also brought to mind the extent to which informed consent and liability play a role in public policy. In the early application of informed consent as it relates to vaccinations, there seemed to be ethical disagreements about how parents should be properly informed about medical warnings for vaccinations. These uncertainties seemed to have increased the number of lawsuits by parents who may not have been properly informed about the adverse effects of some vaccinations. Such lawsuits eventually brought about the need for a federally mandated act and program for compensation. The lack of proper informed consent has also affected clinical trials that include vulnerable populations. These articles helped me become more aware that there is a link between unethical clinical trials and improperly informing participants of adverse risks to vaccinations. This common thread is that if vulnerable populations are not properly informed (even through surrogates), then formal compensation bodies (such as federally mandated programs) should be considered in order to compensate patients or study participants for medical wrongdoings.

Obiora N. Anekwe
Essay 5

In reading the comparative articles on patient advocacy and fiduciary responsibility by Lisa M. Rasmussen and Jeffrey P. Spike, respectfully, I learned more about the balance clinical ethics consultants must maintain in representing patient needs and concerns versus what is viewed as ethical in clinical practice. Patient advocacy seems to be an aspect of bioethics that some in the field are hesitant to embrace. It seems that this resistance stems from the belief that it is inappropriate for clinical ethics consultants to be labeled as advocates for patients when their role should be neutral and unbiased. Both authors explored this particular theme in one way or another, but it is my opinion that patient advocacy, as a means for medical justice in health-care practice, is more pertinent than ever.

It gravely concerns me that medical justice is not explored as much as it should be when so many unethical clinical trials have been conducted in the name of enhancing the greater good. But throughout the tenure of unethical clinical trials, very few seem to advocate for the disenfranchised, even when such patients need someone within the medical and health care community to do so.

During the Christmas holiday season, I read *The Immortal Life of Henrietta Lacks,* by Rebecca Skloot, which chronicles the unethical extraction for research of Henrietta Lacks's cells without her full medical consent. It is my contention that Mrs. Lacks needed someone within the medical community to be her advocate and inform her of her patient rights after her cells were extracted from her body without her permission.

Even though the role of clinical ethics consultants was nonexistent during the 1940s and 1950s when Mrs. Lacks lived, a clinical ethics consultant still may not have advocated for her because they are also accountable to other constituents such as hospitals.

Therefore, a clinical ethics consultant may not have met the full medical needs of Mrs. Lacks, who represented for many, those in the greatest plight. As I reflect upon the two articles I read, I wonder if clinical ethics consultants can truly be employed by the hospital and still represent the patient, even if it is contrary to the values or ethics of their employer. Could such a relationship be a conflict of interest in and of itself? It could easily be recommended as a solution that clinical ethics consultants be employed by independent bodies or advocacy agencies, rather than by the hospitals in which they serve, in order to allow them to fairly and justly advocate and speak independently for patients' medical concerns.

Neither author of the two articles focused on the disenfranchised and other people who cannot advocate for themselves. The poor and disenfranchised cannot even afford the level of health care at which they would encounter clinical ethics consultants. If consultants were independently employed through an advocacy organization, I believe that the poor and disenfranchised, such as Mrs. Lacks, would be provided greater honesty, truth, and medical justice.

But the larger question that should be asked is why cannot clinical ethics consultants be both advocates and a professional clinical ethics consultants? Lisa M. Rasmussen's article, "Patient Advocacy in Clinical Ethics Consultation," raises this very question and argues that it is not that clinical ethics consultants should not also serve as advocates but that it needs to be determined under what conditions they should do so. As I reflect on the clinical discoveries based on the HeLa cells of Henrietta Lacks, I belief that if a clinical ethics consultant had informed her or her family of her medical rights and if doctors had ethical restrictions on their medical practices, then the uninformed extraction of Lacks's cells might not have occurred.

In Jeffrey P. Spike's article, "Do Clinical Ethics Consultants Have a Fiduciary Responsibility to the Patient?" the term *patient advocacy* is replaced with the words, *fiduciary responsibility*. Although the terminology is different, the questions that Jeffrey P. Spike raises are just as pertinent in regard to the systematic role of clinical ethics consultants. As professionals who practices ethics in medicine and health care, clinical ethics consultants have a duty and responsibility to justly meet the needs and concerns of patients in order to preserve their medical rights, which are ethically, legally, and morally binding. As the field of bioethics grows, it is my belief that patient advocacy and fiduciary responsibility will be accepted as norms in the medical and health-care professions.

Obiora N. Anekwe
Essay 6

In reading the article, "New System for Patients to Report Medical Mistakes," by Robert Pear, I found striking correlations between the medical mistakes he discusses and my own research on uninformed consent. The article examined a very comprehensive initiative proposed by the Obama administration in order to report medical errors that currently occur in medical facilities. Specifically, the initiative would focus on medical errors conducted by medical doctors, hospitals, and pharmacists. The reporting of these errors would be facilitated through a customer safety reporting system for patient safety. The Obama administration envisions that the new reporting safety system would be conducted through a website and in telephone interviews. As I read the article, I thought about the unethical clinical trials and experiments that were conducted and financially sponsored by the federal government. The US Public Health Service initiated many of these clinical trials during an era when the eugenics movement was viewed as a justification for conducting unethical research studies. There were no advocates for the patients who participated in these trials. Rather, it was the federal government itself that sponsored these studies for the betterment and medical good of society.

It would have been helpful to many patients who were unjustly sterilized or experimented upon in the past to have had a system in place in order to report medical wrongdoings. Rather than state and federal governments working for medical good for patient care, they instead worked without regard for the detriment and harm of vulnerable women and men. For instance, in Tuskegee, Alabama, African-American men were not treated for syphilis in a forty-year clinical trial. The Tuskegee Syphilis Study was a race-based experiment in order to measure the long-term effects of the nontreatment of syphilis. These men were not informed that they had syphilis and that they were not being treated for the disease. In North Carolina, many women were sterilized by public health officials because these women were viewed as unfit, by traditional standards, to have children. In many instances, these women were sterilized without their permission. They were essentially stripped of their human right to reproduce. These acts were not medical errors or mistakes, but rather, intentional acts of medical wrongdoing that were viewed as the norm by the medical community.

In reflecting on how a medical reporting system could have assisted the vulnerable populations I have described above, I also have to be aware that the medical regulations and laws that exist today did not exist when many of these unethical acts were committed. In my opinion, what is now proposed by the Obama administration to assist patients who have had a medical error imposed upon them is critical to the progress of health care in America.

In order to move forward from past unethical clinical trials, I argue that the proposed federally mandated reporting system also needs to be in place for patients who are participants in studies that may be unethical. Although ethical guidelines are now in place to protect human subjects in research, the proposed reporting system by the Obama administration could include the reporting of medical harm (errors) and wrongdoing by researchers who conduct unethical studies. This would serve as a protective barrier and additional assurance to patients that they would not be taken advantage of or taken for granted. I feel that the Obama administration's proposal will bring to light medical mistakes that are happening today. Unfortunately, it cannot right the wrongs done to so many patients who have been victims to past unethical medical acts, but it can surely make the future better.

Reference

Pear, R. (2012, September 22). New system for patients to report medical mistakes. *The New York Times*. Retrieved from http://www.nytimes.com/2012/09/23/health/new-system-for-patients-to-report-medical-mistakes.htm

Medical Error
Obiora N. Anekwe

A medical wrong can be intentional or inadvertent on the part of a medical or health-care practitioner. The term *medical error* can refer to a multiplicity of unethical acts focused on doctor liability and/or improper or unethical medical practice. Our readings on medical error mostly related to medical procedures or clinical practices involving improper or unethical medical practice. But there is one clinical trial in particular that focuses on a form of medical error known as uninformed consent. Although the Tuskegee Syphilis Study was not highlighted in this week's readings, I suspect that it still serves as a congruent example of intentional medical error, both historically and practically.

The Tuskegee Syphilis Study (1932–1972) is known as the longest clinical trial sponsored by the US federal government. It also represents an example of medical error imposed upon a segmented population of individuals who were purposely left uninformed that they had syphilis. The intent of the syphilis study was to measure the long-term effects of syphilis in the African-American male body. The hypothesis of the study was that the black male body would react to syphilis differently and, therefore, be more resistant to the disease. And the clinical researchers involved in the syphilis study decided to put their theory to practice.

For forty years, the African-American males involved in the study were given placebo drugs and painful spinal taps for treatment, but not beneficial drugs such as penicillin. As a result, many African-American males who were research subjects died due to nonmedical treatment, medical deception, and medical error. Although public health officials who conducted the study deceived the men through recruitment flyers, a lack of informed patient consent, and just blatant lies to patients that they were being treated for their "bad blood," doctors still believed that they were conducting their research for the greater medical good.

As a result of these unjust, immoral, and unethical acts by medical officials, the men involved in the Tuskegee Syphilis Study decided to file a joint lawsuit against the federal government in 1973. The lawsuit, *Charlie W. Pollard, el al. v. United States of America, et al* (1973), was settled out of court, which brought forth monetary and policy benefits for the men who suffered unjustly from their uninformed participation in the Tuskegee Syphilis Study. However, many family members of these men still believe that full reconciliation for the medical errors which affected their loved ones has not been provided. These medical acts affected the physical, psychological, and spiritual aspects of the men and their family members. For instance, many wives of the victims involved in the Tuskegee Syphilis Study were also infected with syphilis because their husbands were unaware that they had the disease. This affected the physical and mental well-being of their offspring as well.

As an emerging bioethicist, I believe we should be aware of unethical studies, such as the Tuskegee Syphilis Study, because if we are unaware, similar studies may be repeated. Whether intentional or not, such unethical behavior still has grave consequences. We must be willing to recognize this fact and try our best to invest in medical research that does not bring shame to the field of bioethics. Let this process begin with us.

Was the Tuskegee Syphilis Study a Form of Medical Error or Something Much Worse?
Ejinkonye C. Anekwe

The Tuskegee Syphilis Study was considered a form of medical error for a multitude of reasons. First, the practitioners of the study did not inform the prospective patients about the risks involved in the study. Because of this omission, the patients were unaware that they were even part of a study. Second, there was no treatment given in the study. Without treatment, the patients died from the natural progression of syphilis. These individuals were not even told they had syphilis; rather, they were told that they had "bad blood," a colloquial expression encompassing a number of diseases that affected the bloodstream in the human body. Third, the doctors abused the patients' bodies through painfully invasive spinal taps, which today would be considered malpractice. If doctors today employed the same tactics that were used during the Tuskegee Syphilis Study, they would find themselves in front of a medical review board, and subsequently have their medical licenses revoked.

Was the Tuskegee Syphilis Study worse than a series of medical errors? In most respects, it was. One factor was scientific racism. The study was performed against a backdrop of intense racism. During the beginnings of the study, many scientists thought African-Americans and other minorities were physiologically different from Caucasians. The belief did not stop at skin color. For instance, there was an assumption that African-Americans were impervious to pain, as well as some illnesses. In addition, the scientists and doctors involved in the Tuskegee Syphilis Study believed that bodies of African-Americans handled syphilis better than Caucasians. Today, scientists consider those ideas not just antiquated, but nonsense. Since the Human Genome Project concluded in 2005, scientists now know that there is no genetic basis for race. In other words, all humans living on Earth are of the same species, *Homo sapiens*. There is only one race, which is the human race. Unfortunately, in 1932, most people could not fathom that notion. Because of this ignorance, hundreds of men were made to suffer.

Another factor that made the Tuskegee Syphilis Study worse than simple malpractice was the denial of treatment. If medical mistakes were made, why didn't doctors switch to penicillin to treat syphilis after understanding their mistakes? That act alone would have saved the remaining patients and offered a modicum of credibility for the project. The intention was never to treat these men for syphilis. Rather, the intent of the study was to see the effects of syphilis in African-American males to the very end—in other words, to the end of the patients' lives. To put it succinctly, the doctors watched the patients die. It was as if someone was watching a murder in progress and did not call 911 because he or she wanted the person to die.

Human experimentation is meant to help people. Yes, there are risks involved, but those risks must be implicitly written and explained to the patients. If the patients cannot read or write, then the instructions and risks should be read to the patients. The researchers in the Tuskegee Syphilis Study did not intend for patients to be informed about their rights, however limited those rights were in 1930s Alabama. In conclusion, the study was conducted with the intent to use a subset of the population in order to study the natural progression of syphilis. The intent was not to treat them, because such treatment would undermine the very purpose of the study. Thus, the practices employed in the study were much worse than medical error.

The History of Syphilis and Early Research on its Effects on the Human Body
Ejinkonye C. Anekwe

Introduction
The disease of syphilis is classified as a *Treponema* species. This species includes yaws, pinta, venereal syphilis, and endemic (nonvenereal) syphilis, according to the 1988 article "Origin and Antiquity of Syphilis: Paleopathological Diagnosis and Interpretation" by Baker et al. All four of these diseases, collectively known as treponematosis, are caused by *Treponema pallidum* (Baker et al, 1988, p. 704). The origins of syphilis are clear.

Baker et al (1988), citing Hudson (1963a, 1965a), state that syphilis originated during the Paleolithic period in sub-Saharan Africa as yaws, a childhood disease. Yaws is spread through dermal contact between people, and migrated with hunter-gatherer groups (Baker et al, 1988, p. 704). By the time these groups settled in drier climates, syphilis was limited to the groin, mouth, and armpits (Baker et al, 1988, p. 704). As humans settled into larger, Neolithic cities, syphilis, especially in the form of yaws, spread through the population.

As humans started to build cities around 4,000 BC, personal hygiene improved due to access to clean water, exercise of regular bathing practices, and proper accommodations. As such, the cases of endemic syphilis decreased among children. According to Baker, citing Hudson (1965a), humans began to grow up without previous exposure to syphilis, thus only contracting the disease through sexual contact. As a result, the venereal form of syphilis was spread through sexual intercourse, including prostitution and promiscuity (Baker et al, 1988, p. 704).

Syphilis, yaws, and leprosy used to be grouped in the same category in ancient times (Baker et al, 1988, p. 704). However, these diseases are different in their presentation and symptoms. For instance, Baker et al (1988), citing Olansky (1981), state that syphilis (venereal) can incubate for ten to ninety days before it appears as primary lesions in the anus and genitals. The lesions that are secondary appear on the mucous membranes and the skin (Baker et al, 1988, p. 704). Before the use of penicillin, syphilis occurred in 5 percent of adult city dwellers (Baker et al, 1988, p. 704). Syphilis can also spread in bone tissue. According to Baker et al (1988), citing prepenicillin data compiled by Steinbock (1976), 10–20 percent of all syphilis cases involve skeletal lesions. However, bone lesions went undetected in patients with early stages of syphilis (Baker et al, 1988, p. 704).

Theories Regarding Transmission of Syphilis

The theories regarding transmission of syphilis in both Europe and the New World are controversial. The most common school of thought was that syphilis was brought from the New World to Europe by Christopher Columbus and his crew in 1493 (Baker et al, 1988, p. 703). Afterward, from the late 1490s to around 1500, a syphilis outbreak ravaged the European continent, and at that time, Europeans did not have immunity to the New World form of syphilis (Baker et al 1988, p. 703). Another hypothesis suggests that, rather than being a new disease in Europe, syphilis was already present in Europe and was classified as a form of leprosy. It was not until the onset of the epidemic in the 1490s that syphilis was classified as a separate disease (Baker et al, 1988, p. 703). At this point, syphilis became known as a *Treponema* species. The cases of syphilis were relatively low due to small numbers of people. As populations increased, syphilis cases increased, particularly with dermal contact between children (Baker et al, 1988, p. 703). In addition, a third theory states that syphilis strains developed independently in both Europe and the Americas (Baker et al, 1988, p. 704). The different types of treponematosis manifestations depended on the biological makeup of the environment (Baker et al, 1988, p. 704).

Early Study and Treatment of Syphilis

Syphilis used to be an enigmatic disease. Throughout the nineteenth century, the disease was mysterious enough to give rise to myths and superstitions of all types. For instance, Laura Englestein (1986) mentioned that several myths and rumors were generated by lack of knowledge concerning sexual transmission of syphilis. This misinformation was spread by doctors themselves (Engelstein, 1986, p. 1036). During the Victorian Era, there were no clinical trials for determining the transmission and subsequent spread of syphilis. In the absence of these trials, nonscientific judgments about syphilis led to what Engelstein called "an exaggerated notion on the incidence of syphilis and confusion about how the disease really spread." She goes on to point out that, "This led the public to believe that one could contract syphilis through nonsexual contact" (1986, p. 1036). It was not until later in the nineteenth century that syphilis would begin to be thoroughly researched.

Another aspect of syphilis transmission was the concept of race and class. For instance, Victorian-era doctors believed that syphilis could be transmitted through nonvenereal and venereal means. While nonvenereal means of transmission involved touching, breastfeeding, and contact with inanimate objects, venereal transmission dealt with sexual contact (Engelstein, 1986, pp. 1036–1037). In terms of sexual contact, doctors during Victorian times believed that moral decay among lower-class individuals was the main cause of syphilis epidemics (Engelstein, 1986, p. 1037). Syphilis was thought to be traced specifically to the nineteenth century urban dweller. Bachelors and prostitutes in cities were blamed for syphilitic outbreaks (Engelstein, 1986, p. 1037). Moreover, many people in the nineteenth century also believed that syphilis was prevalent in nonvenereal form among *less civilized* people in Norway, Sweden, and Lithuania, which were poor countries during that time period. African-Americans were also thought to harbor the nonvenereal form (Engelstein, 1986, p. 1037). These racist assumptions regarding disease would persist into the twentieth century.

Origins of the Tuskegee Syphilis Study

The study of syphilis in the early twentieth century was overshadowed by racial assumptions that have now been discredited by modern science and medicine. In fact, the results of the Tuskegee Syphilis Study were published by J. K. Schafer in 1954. Reading this article was chilling because it was written approximately twenty years after the initiation of the study. Shafer et al (1954) discussed the need for research into the lifespan of people afflicted with syphilis. The researchers explained that a need for a national venereal disease control program arose out of epidemic levels of syphilis in the United States. Syphilis was said to be the number one cause of rejection of draftees during World War I (Shafer et al, 1954, p. 235). Thus, something needed to be done to reduce the number of syphilis cases nationwide.

The question posed in the article was the effects of syphilis on life expectancy (Shafer et al, 1954, p. 235). In other words, the researchers wanted to know the natural progression of the disease. They knew that syphilis had a life span of two years, with chronic symptoms that persist up to twenty years, but few data shed light on the natural course of the disease in people (Shafer et al, 1954, p. 235).

A European study that involved the monitoring of untreated syphilis patients was the Norway study. Shafer and his colleagues stated that the results of the experiment, known as the Bruusgaard Study, were available as of 1929. In the study, Dr. Boeck, the head of the Dermatology and Syphilology Clinic at the University of Oslo, treated 2,181 people with syphilis at its early phase. The patients were placed in the hospital and were given treatments that helped ease their symptoms (Shafer et al, 1954, p. 235). However, Dr. Boeck did not treat them with arsenic or mercury, even though they were available. Bruusgaard, the namesake of the study, analyzed a group of 473 syphilitic patients to determine if they lived up to forty years after treatment. According to the analysis conducted by Bruusgaard, 164 of the 473 patients died, while 309 lived. Out of the 473 patients, 27.7 percent were free of syphilitic symptoms (Shafer et al, 1954, p. 236). However, the Bruusgaard Study was criticized for its lack of accuracy in the diagnosis and treatment of syphilis and for the lack of long-term study of populations (Shafer et al, 1954, p. 236).

The Bruusgaard Study of Norway did provide researchers with some degree of analysis regarding the treatment of syphilis. However, researchers wanted a study that examined the accurate life expectancy of syphilitic patients over a long period of time. In particular, there was a desire to ascertain the effects of the venereal disease in shortening life expectancy (Shafer et al, 1954, p. 237). There seemed to be interest in distinguishing the effects of syphilis among different ethnicities, namely African-Americans and whites. Previous results published by the Cooperate Clinical Studies in 1937 used a theoretical life table of males with syphilis. The results, which studied life expectancy among syphilitic males, indicated that among adult males thirty to sixty years old, African-American life expectancy decreased by 30 percent, which was greater than the 17 percent drop in life expectancy due to syphilis (Shafer et al, 1954, p. 237). The results of that study were used as a basis for the Tuskegee Syphilis Study.

Throughout the early part of the twentieth century, health conditions in the Southern United States indicated that syphilis was at epidemic levels among African-Americans. Studies conducted by the Rosenwald and Rockefeller Foundations confirmed this (Shafer et al, 1954, p. 237). One southern county in particular had a high number of syphilitic cases among African-Americans. The county in particular, Macon County, was home to Tuskegee Institute (now Tuskegee University). The foundations, along with the United States Public Health Service, sought to diagnose and treat syphilis in the South. These entities also wanted to study untreated syphilis in the African-American male (Shafer et al, 1954, p. 237).

The reason for choosing only males was that there would be no problems with syphilis being transmitted congenitally (Shafer et al, 1954, p. 237). Another reason for the choice was that the researchers wanted to choose patients from the same age and socio-economic background. An African-American nurse was selected to monitor the progress of the group, which included patients who were afflicted with syphilis as well as patients who were nonsyphilitic. The nurse was required to report her findings to a health officer located in the same area (Shafer et al, 1954, p. 237).

When patients died from syphilis, the bodies were to be used for postmortem analysis. Funding for these autopsies was granted by the Milbank Memorial Fund (Shafer et al, 1954, p. 238). The bodies were shipped to National Institutes of Health of the Public Health Service, more specifically, the Division of Pathology. Even though some patients moved to the North, there were still enough bodies to conduct autopsies (Shafer et al, 1954, p. 238).

Shafer and his colleagues gave very detailed descriptions of the manner in which the study was conducted. For instance, 408 untreated syphilis patients and 192 patients without syphilis were selected. What was more shocking was that of the 408 original syphilitic patients selected between 1932 and 1933, 165, or 40.4 percent, died. In addition, fifty-one of the nonsyphilis patients, or 26.6 percent, died during the study (Shafer et al, 1954, p. 238). Sixty percent of the deceased patients were given autopsies (Shafer et al, 1954, p. 238).

The results of the Shafer study indicated that the greatest numbers of mortality among syphilitic patients occurred among men between twenty-five and seventy-four years of age. In addition, there were 17 percent more deaths among untreated syphilitic men between twenty-five and fifty than among all men in the nonsyphilitic group (Shafer et al, 1954, p. 240).

Conclusion

The Shafer study exemplified the attitudes of the early twentieth century toward patients, especially African-Americans. Because the Norwegian Bruusgaard Study was not very conclusive, researchers in the United States Public Health Service, along with wealthy foundations, wanted to reduce epidemic levels of syphilis in the South. However, the researchers did not give treatment to the patients in the study. They simply let them die. Today, such attitudes would be considered antiquated at best inhumane at worst. In closing, the Shafer study was basically the blueprint for the Tuskegee Syphilis Study. It was by no means the only study, but it was a detailed study. It is also an example of how not to conduct an experiment.

References

Baker, B., Armelagos, G., Becker, M., Brothwell, D., Drusini, A., Geise, M., Kelley, M., Moritoto, I., Morris, I., Nurse, G., Powell, M., Rothschild, B., and Saunders, S. (1988). "Origin and Antiquity of Syphilis: Paleopathological Diagnosis and Interpretation (and Comments and Reply)." *Current Anthropology,* 29(5), 703–737. Retrieved from http:www.jstor.org/stable/2743609

Engelstein, L. (1986). "Syphilis, Historical and Actual: Cultural Geography of a Disease." *Reviews of Infectious Diseases,* 8(6), 1036–1048. Retrieved from http:www.jstor.org/stable/4453996

Shafer, J.K., Usilton, L., Gleeson, G., and Buncher, C. "Untreated Syphilis in the Male Negro" (1954) [with Commentary]. *Public Health Reports (1974), 121,* Supplement 1: Historical Collection 1878–2005 (2006), pp. 234–241. Retrieved from http://www.jstor.org/stable/20057073

The Massacre of the Herero in Namibia
Ejinkonye C. Anekwe

Introduction

Before the Nazi Party came to power in Germany, that country was a colonial power in Africa. In Namibia, the German colonial administration was responsible for the destruction of most of the Herero ethnic group. The purpose of this essay is to point out the origins of Nazi human experimentation and to understand how the German colonial experiences in Namibia contributed to the implementation of the final solution. The author will discuss the oppression and plight of the Herero people, followed by their near extermination by German colonial authorities. The author will also present information on early human experimentation on Africans at concentration camps throughout Namibia, even though these accounts are limited. The goal of writing the essay is to inform the reader about the nascent attempts at experimentation as a means of perpetuating racial stereotypes.

The Plight of the Herero People under German Colonial Rule

Namibia was once a colonial possession of Germany. The German authorities intended to turn Namibia (then called Southwest Africa) into a settlers' colony with Africans forming the bulk of the servant class (Adhikiri, 2008, p. 305). The African population, known as *natives*, was punished severely for the minutest things. The use of corporal punishment was common among the African population (Adhikiri, 2008, p. 306). As far as the Germans were concerned, the Africans were inferior to Europeans. The African population, especially the Herero and Nama ethnic groups, were frustrated with being treated as virtual slaves. The Herero were Bantu people from the middle of Namibia, while the Nama were Hottentot people from Southern Namibia. Both groups were small, with eighty thousand Herero and twenty thousand Nama. The numbers of Herero people could have even been as high as eighty-five thousand (Pennington and Harpending, 1991, p. 210). Both were cattle herders and were armed with rifles (Abagond, 2012). In 1904, the Herero and Nama decided to take matters into their own hands.

German-Herero War of 1904

The Herero rebelled against the German colonial government in January 1904. The Germans were initially outnumbered by the Herero and Nama (Abagond. 2012). The African rebellion was actually gaining strength, but by August of 1904, the

Germans defeated them (Pennington and Harpending, 1991, p. 210). With the Germans bogged down with fighting the Nama, Lieutenant General Lothario bin Trotha was ordered to suppress the Herero rebellion. With cannons and machine guns, von Trotha defeated the Herero (Abagond, 2012). However, the Germans were not simply satisfied with victory. Over the next four years, 80 percent of the Herero and half of the Nama were killed as part of a planned genocide by the German government (Adhikari, 2008, p. 303). The Herero massacre was considered the first genocide of the twentieth century (Adhikari, 2008, p. 303). The genocide and its aftermath are well documented by the perpetrators (the Germans), the victims (the Herero and Nama peoples), and academics. According to Adhikari (2008), the genocide was planned well in advance of the Herero defeat. For instance, von Trotha, who headed the German army in Namibia, promulgated an order to exterminate the Herero in October of 1904. The Vernichtungsbefehl (extermination order) stated that since the Herero were no longer part of Germany, they were required to vacate Namibia. Von Trotha also said that any Herero who did not leave the colony would be killed on sight (Adhikari, 2008, p. 304). Many Herero escaped into neighboring countries, such as Botswana. Pennington and Harpending (1991) conducted research into the remaining numbers of Herero people in Botswana. After the war, fifteen thousand to twenty-five thousand Herero remained in Namibia out of a pre-war population approaching eighty-five thousand (Pennington and Harpending, 1991, p. 210). Both researchers stated that the number of Herero who escaped to Botswana was undetermined. What is known, however, is that the Herero were chased out of Namibia by German patrols (Pennington and Harpending, 1991, p. 210). Many ended up in the desert wastelands (Gewald, 1999, p. 21). There, the Herero died of thirst (BBC, 2011). The remainder were forbidden to own land or cattle. Some were even forced to work for German settlers or shipped off to work in South African mines (Gewald, 1999, p. 22). The Nama were next, with German troops fighting Nama guerrillas in skirmishes. Eventually, ten thousand Nama were massacred, which was half of the twenty thousand Nama present during the late 1800s (Abagond, 2012).

What happened to the Herero who remained in Namibia? Many were either killed by German patrols or sent to concentration camps such as Shark Island. When von Trotha lifted the extermination order in December 1904, the Herero survivors were sent to concentration camps (Adhikari, 2008, p. 311). Some Herero were taken from the deserts (two which they had escaped) to camps along the cold coastline. Some were even tricked by missionaries into believing that they were being offered sanctuary and food, only to be placed in these death camps (Adhikari, 2008, p. 311). The German authorities felt that the concentration camps were needed in order to cleanse Namibia of the Herero. In fact, von Trotha believed that he did the right thing by referring to all African tribes as inferior. He also felt that the Herero should be eliminated in Namibia. This coincided with the social Darwinists' beliefs in the conquest of what the Germans thought were racially inferior tribes (Adhikari, 2008, p. 305). Adhikari stated that social Darwinism advocates not only conquest but the total replacement of one group with another group (Adhikiri, 2008, p. 305). As a result, von Trotha ordered the surviving Herero into various concentration camps. Some of these camps were located on the cold, Namibian coast. Camps such as those at Swakopmund and Luderitz were known for their high casualty rate because of the Herero's unusual exposure to the cold. Deaths were also caused by whippings, poor and inadequate diet, and overwork. In the Swakopmund concentration camp, 40 percent of the prisoners died in February 1905 (Adhikari, 2008, p. 312). These camps operated from January 1905 to January 1908, the month of the Kaiser's birthday (Adhikari, 2008, p. 311).

One infamous camp was Shark Island. It is known as the world's first death camp and the harshest (Adhikari, 2008, p. 313). Located in Southern Namibia, the island is subjected to icy winds (Adhikari, 2008, p. 312). The Herero were given very little clothing, and their shelter consisted of simple wood huts. The prisoners were made to perform back-breaking, menial work on the camp's pier and other projects. This led to a 70 percent mortality rate among the prisoners at Shark Island, satisfying the intent of the German authorities to kill off the Herero through neglect and overwork (Adhikari, 2008, p. 313).

In addition to the deaths at Shark Island and other concentration camps, human experiments occurred among the prisoners. Although there is a dearth of data regarding the extent of experimentations, books and films discuss the forced sterilization of African women in Namibia and, later, in Nazi Germany. Delroy Constantine-Sims, of the University of Essex, wrote an informative essay on the BBC documentary, *Hitler's Forgotten Victims*. The film explores, among other things, the roots of German racism toward Africans. In the essay, Constantine-Sims discussed how after the massacre of the Herero in 1904, some Herero were subjected to experiments. In addition, Africans were forcibly sterilized to prevent miscegenation between Germans and Africans (Constantine-Simms, 1997). Eugen Fischer, a doctor, supervised the sterilization program in Namibia. Later, in Nazi Germany, Fischer, as a senior geneticist, would lead the effort to sterilize African women residing there (Constantine-Simms, 1997). Other experiments involved the collection of skulls for use in race-based experiments in Germany. These experiments were meant to prove that Africans were inferior to Europeans (BBC, 2012). As of 2011, only twenty of the skulls were returned to Namibia. The rest languish in storage in Germany (BBC, 2011).

Conclusion

The use (or abuse) of Africans as virtual slaves and, eventually, test subjects may have been a precursor to the larger holocaust that happened forty years later. The Herero never received an apology nor reparation payments from Germany for the genocide. Germany instead stated that, while they regret what happened, the German government already gave $173 million in aid to Namibia for 2011–2012. The effects of the Herero genocide still resonate in Namibia, with the German minority owning land taken from the Herero, while many Africans remain without land (BBC, 2012). Also, there are no monuments to the thousands of Herero and Nama people who died in the concentration camps of Namibia (BBC, 2012). Please keep in mind that in much of Africa, land ownership is a significant source of wealth. Without land, a person is poor. Thus, the author can imagine how frustrating it is to get the African population in Namibia to receive recognition for being victims of genocide. The families of the Tuskegee Syphilis Study participants went through the same struggle to get an apology from the United States government. For the Namibian victims, the experimentation with their skulls is indicative of scientific racism. As in the Tuskegee Syphilis Study, there was great effort by the German government to prove that Africans were not as intelligent as Europeans. Today, scientists refer to these racist ideas as pseudoscience. However, the damage done to generations of African victims will take many years to undo.

References

Abagond. (2012). The Herero and Nama genocide. Retrieved from http://abagond.wordpress.com/2012/07/26/the-herero-and-nama-genocide/

Adhikari, M. (2008). "'Streams of blood and streams of money: Streams of blood and streams of money': New perspectives on the annihilation of the Herero and Nama peoples of Namibia, 1904–1908," *Kronos*, 34, 303–320. Retrieved from http://www.jstor.org/stable/41056613

BBC.com. (2011). "Remembering German crimes in Namibia." BBC. Retrieved from http://www.bbc.co.uk/news/world-africa-15257857

Gewald, J. B. (1999). "The Road of the Man Called Love and the Sack of Sero: The HereroGerman War and the Export of Herero Labour to the South African Rand," *The Journal of African History*, 40(1), 21–40. Retrieved from http://www.jstor.org/stable/183393

Pennington, R. and Harpending, H. (1991). "How Many Refugees Were There? History and Population Change Among the Herero and Mbanderu of Northwestern Botswana," Botswana Notes and Records, 23, 209–221. Retrieved from http://www.jstor.org/stable/40980852. Accessed: 05/03/2013 11:11

CHAPTER 4:

PATHWAYS TO HEALING: STORIES OF REDEMPTION AND RECONCILIATION

Uninformed Consent: The US Public Health Study of Untreated Syphilis in the Negro Male (1932–1972), Macon County Alabama
Obiora N. Anekwe

A Definition of Informed Consent

Informed consent usually refers to consent that a person gives that meets certain minimum standards. Further, an informed consent can be given based upon a clear understanding of the facts, implications, and future consequences of an action. In order to provide informed consent, the person involved in a study must have adequate reasoning faculties and be in possession of relevant facts at the time consent is given (Berg, Appelbaum, Parker, and Lidz, 2001). Impairments in reasoning and judgment such as basic intellectual/emotional immaturity, high levels of stress, severe mental illness, intoxication, severe sleep deprivation, Alzheimer's disease, or being in a coma constitute examples of impaired consent. The term *informed consent* was first used in a 1957 medical malpractice case by attorney Paul G. Gebhard (Solomon, 2006).

Informed consent is also defined as the procedure whereby patients consent to or refuse a medical intervention based on information provided by a health-care professional regarding the nature and potential consequences of the proposed medical treatment in a health-care setting (Coy, 1989). One goal of informed consent is to help patients make decisions about their medical care (Coy, 1989). Informed consent may be documented through a written consent using a template prepared by the Human Participants Review Committee and signed by the participant or his or her legally authorized representative. A copy of the informed consent document must be given to the person who signed the agreement (Tuskegee University Manual for Institutional Review Board, 2005). Two types of informed consent agreements are permissible for the researcher to obtain: 1) a written informed consent agreement that includes all of the basic elements of informed consent and 2) an oral informed consent agreement which consists of a script of the information presented verbally and a short consent form that states that the elements of informed consent have been presented orally to the participant and that a witness was present (Tuskegee University Manual for Institutional Review Board, 2005).

There are several exceptions to requirements for informed consent. The Human Participants Review Committee (HPRC) may approve a consent procedure that does not include, or which alters, some or all of the elements of informed consent, or they may waive the requirements to obtain informed consent, provided the HPRC finds and documents the following:

1. The research involves no more than minimal risk.

2. The rights and welfare of participants will not be adversely affected.

3. The research could not practically be carried out without the waiver or alteration.

4. Whenever appropriate, the participants will be provided with additional pertinent information after participation.

5. Or the research or demonstrations project is to be conducted by, or subject to approval of, state or local government officials and is designed to study, evaluate, or examine public benefit or service programs or proposed changes in programs, procedures, methods or levels of payment (Tuskegee University Manual for Institutional Review Board, 2005).

As indicated in the Tuskegee University Manual for Institutional Review, informed consent is necessary for all research and other activities that involve human participants. Informed consent is the process of voluntary agreement based upon adequate knowledge and understanding of relevant information germane to participating in research (Tuskegee University Manual for Institutional Review Board, 2005). The investigator may determine, within the limits of this policy, which method would best serve the interests of the subject population of the particular project. However, the Human Participants Review Committee reserves the right, upon review of the research, to require alternate and/or more stringent means of securing consent if necessary in order to protect the participant(s) (Tuskegee University Manual for Institutional Review Board, 2005). If the participants are not able to provide personal consent, for reasons such as age, mental state, legal or other such status, then permission must be granted from the parent(s) or a legal guardian, and assent must be secured from the participant who is a minor (Tuskegee University Manual for Institutional Review Board, 2005).

Two ethical principles serve as the moral foundation of informed consent: the Principle of Autonomy and the Principle of Beneficence. These two principles often lead to conflicting conceptions of informed consent (Coy, 1989). The Principle of

Beneficence is used as a moral foundation of informed consent; the patient's consent is obtained in order to protect the patient's interests by helping to ensure the best medical outcome for the patient (Coy, 1989). When treatment can potentially harm a patient, informed consent is necessary because of a potential harm to the patient (Coy, 1989). On the other hand, with respect to the Principle of Autonomy, the patient's right to self-determination is of primary importance. When this principle serves as the moral foundation of informed consent, consent is required because it helps protect a person's right to self-determination (Coy, 1989).

Some medical acts cannot legally take place, because of lack of informed consent. In cases in which a person is unable to provide informed consent, another person is authorized to give consent on a patient or subject's behalf (Dunn, Nowrangi, Palmer, Jeste, and Saks, 2006). In cases where a research participant is provided insufficient information to formulate an informed decision, significant ethical issues can arise. In such cases in a clinical trial setting, these ethical issues are prevented through an ethical committee known as the Institutional Review Board (IRB) (Fisher, 2006).

Research Study Background

According to Arthur L. Caplan (1992), the US Public Health Study of Untreated Syphilis in the Negro Male, 1932–1972 (also known as the Tuskegee Syphilis Study or the Tuskegee Experiment) is the longest nontherapeutic experiment on human beings in medical history. The Tuskegee Syphilis Study was based on a study of nearly two thousand untreated syphilitics in Oslo, Norway, from 1891 to 1910 that was published with a follow-up study in 1929 (Standler, 1997). The study held in Tuskegee, Macon County, Alabama, which was initiated by the United States Public Health Service in 1932, was designed to determine the natural course of untreated latent syphilis in 399 African-American men. These 399 research participants with syphilis were matched against 201 uninfected African-American men who served as a control group. The infected men were not fully informed that they had syphilis (Centers for Disease Control and Prevention, 2011). Rather, they were informed that they were being treated for "bad blood," a local term in the Macon County area that described several illnesses such as syphilis, anemia, and fatigue (Centers for Disease Control and Prevention, 2011).

The research subjects were recruited through deception by promises of special treatment for "bad blood." These treatments were spinal taps (painful lumbar punctures) done without anesthesia to study the neurological effects of syphilis without the research subjects' informed consent (Standler, 1997). The treatments actually induced further pain and caused further life altering physical damage to many research study subjects.

The Role of Government and Other Institutions

The true nature of the syphilis study was kept from the research subjects in order to ensure their full cooperation. The benefits of participation in the study included "free medical treatment," a proper burial after death, and a small allowance for participation. The local African-American and white physicians in Macon County, Alabama, and surrounding counties were recruited by the USPHS officials to withhold treatment from the men with syphilis (Centers for Disease Control and Prevention, 2011). Autopsy and physician assessments were conducted at the John A. Andrew Memorial Hospital on the campus of the Tuskegee Institute (now Tuskegee University), Tuskegee, Alabama. A number of Tuskegee Institute faculty and staff were involved in the study (Centers for Disease Control and Prevention, 2011).

Similar Cases Involving a Breach of Informed Consent

In October 2010, Wellesley College historian and bioethicist, Dr. Susan Reverby, discovered that syphilis experiments were held from 1946 to 1948 by the United States Department of Health in a mental hospital in which American doctors infected prisoners, soldiers, and patients with syphilis and gonorrhea (Smith, 2010). A total number of 696 men and women were exposed to syphilis without their informed consent (Smith, 2010). Once the research participants contracted syphilis or gonorrhea, they were given antibiotics. John Charles Cutler, a public health researcher who worked in the US Public Health Study on Untreated Syphilis in the Negro (also known as the Tuskegee Syphilis Study, 1932–1972), was also involved as a lead researcher in the syphilis study held in Guatemala (Smith, 2010).

Ethical Implications

Although penicillin was found to be an effective treatment for syphilis in the 1940s, the United States Public Health Service (USPHS) purposely allowed the Tuskegee Syphilis Study to continue to take place for an additional twenty-five years among African-American males without treatment by penicillin. The aftermath of the study led to the establishment of the National Commission for the Protection of Human Subjects of Biomedical and Behavioral Research and the National Research Act. The National Research Act (1974) required the establishment of institutional review boards (IRBs) at institutions receiving federal support (Centers for Disease Control and Prevention, 2011). Currently, research studies require informed consent (with exceptions for US federal agencies which can be kept secret by executive order), communication of diagnosis, and accurate reporting of test results.

The Tuskegee Syphilis Study also led to the 1979 Belmont Report and the establishment of the Office for Human Research Protections (OHRP) (Office of Human Research Protections, 2005). Additionally, federal laws and regulations requiring Institutional Review Boards for the protection of human subjects in studies involving human subjects were mandated. The Office for Human Research Protections (OHRP) manages this unit within the US Department of Health and Human Services (HHS) (Office of Human Research Protections, 2008).

Several unethical issues involving human research subjects were highlighted in the Tuskegee Syphilis Study. The first issue, that of informed consent, refers to informing or telling research participants about all aspects of the potential research that may influence their decision to participate. The investigators in the syphilis study took advantage of a population of African-American men who received low levels of care (Heintzelman, 2003). Their interactions with the doctors and nurses were based on their perceptions of them as authority figures who would serve the best interests of the research participants. The United States Public Health Service (USPHS) acted with medical deception in the recruitment of research participants. The USPHS officials did not explain to the subjects that the survey was designed to detect syphilis. For instance, the term "bad blood" was used by the doctors and never defined for the subjects (Heintzelman, 2003). The African-American men in the study were not informed that they had syphilis and they were not provided treatment for the disease. The research subjects trusted the USPHS officials because of the medical authority that they represented through their medical work in the surrounding community.

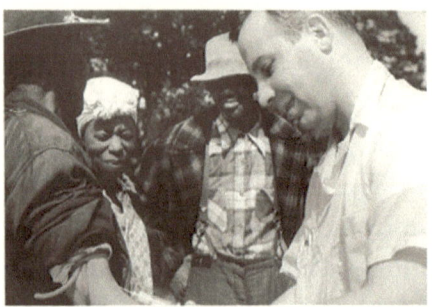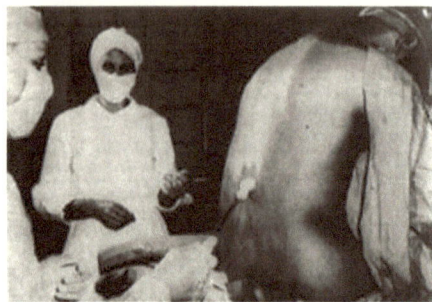

(The left hand picture shows an African-American man having his blood drawn by US public health officials for the testing of syphilis during the Tuskegee Syphilis Study. The right hand picture depicts the spinal tap testing conducted on African-American males during the Tuskegee Syphilis Study.) *Source: The National Archives and Records Administration, Southeast Region, Morrow, Georgia.*

The second unethical action that occurred in the study has to do with the withholding of treatment for research purposes (Heintzelman, 2003). When the syphilis study was evaluated, the researchers judged that the benefits of nontreatment outweighed the benefits of treatment. The research subjects were not provided a choice about continuing participation in the study once penicillin had become available in the 1940s. In fact, the USPHS officials prevented the research subjects from receiving penicillin treatment (Heintzelman, 2003). This decision was based on the quiescent state of the disease, assumptions about the participants, and fear related to the danger of lethal reactions if these men received penicillin. When the syphilis study concluded in 1972, the remaining funds could not be used for penicillin treatment due to the USPHS grant guidelines (Heintzelman, 1996). As bioethicist Dr. Susan E. Lederer noted, the Tuskegee Syphilis Study was a study of undertreated syphilis rather than the study of untreated syphilis, because the USPHS officials enrolled many men who had undergone treatment and there was no written protocol for treatment (The Presidential Commission for the Study of Bioethical Issues, 2011).

Other unethical issues were involved in the Tuskegee Syphilis Study. According to the state law of Alabama in 1972, the reporting and medical treatment of venereal diseases was a state mandated requirement (Heintzelman, 2003). The USPHS officials ignored the state law and chose to disregard the impact of untreated syphilis on the wives and children of the men who were research subjects. Additionally, accurate medical records were not kept by the USPHS. The exact number of African-American men who died from syphilis is not known (Heintzelman, 2003). The number of survivors is estimated to be between seventy-six and 111. The number of those who died was estimated to be between twenty-eight and 101. The last study participant, Mr. Ernest L. Hendon, died at the age of ninety-seven on January 16, 2004 (Centers for Disease Control and Prevention, 2011). By the conclusion of the experiments conducted over a forty-year period, twenty-eight men had died directly due to nontreatment of syphilis, one hundred were dead of related complications, forty of the research participant's wives had been infected with syphilis, and nineteen of their children were born with congenital syphilis (Centers for Disease Control and Protection, 2011).

The personal beliefs within the medical profession about the nature of African-American men and their sexual behavior impacted the outcome of the study (Heintzelman, 2003). The health of the African-American community in Macon County and surrounding areas was, therefore, jeopardized because of the nontreatment of the men who contracted syphilis. Although a comprehensive medical report about the syphilis study was not published, this study was reported in various medical journals for forty years without criticism from the medical establishment (Heintzelman, 2003). The medical doctors involved in the study did not question the morality of the study.

As indicated in Graphic 1, there was a significant lack of informed consent among the African-American men who participated in the Tuskegee Syphilis Study. The lack of moral and ethical policies to guide the study prohibited the implementation of policies that could have prevented the unnecessary deaths of men who contracted syphilis. Health awareness, education on preventive measures, and penicillin treatments for the men could have been effective and ideal in the treatment of syphilis. Instead, the prevention of medical treatment by penicillin and the lack of full disclosure nurtured an environment where secrecy and un-informed consent were pivotal to the sustaining of unfair and unethical health and medical practice.

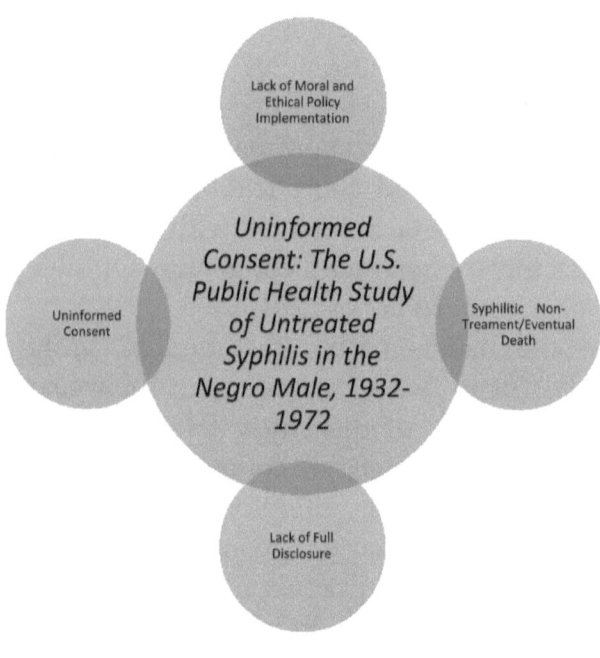

Graphic 1

Research Implications

After the conclusion of the Tuskegee Syphilis Study in 1972, the federal government changed its research practices in order to prevent a similar study from occurring in the future. In 1974, the National Research Act created the National Commission for the Protection of Human Subjects of Biomedical and Behavioral Research (Centers for Disease Control and Prevention, 2011). This group identified the basic principles of research conduct. Voluntary informed consent from research subjects was also mandatory for studies conducted by and/or financially funded by the Department of Health, Education, and Welfare (DHEW). The law also required that DHEW-supported studies that used human subjects had to be reviewed by Institutional Review Boards (IRBs) to determine if the studies meet ethical standards (Centers for Disease Control and Prevention, 2011). Another result of the Tuskegee Syphilis Study was the lifetime medical benefits and burial services to all living study participants. As part of the 1974 legal settlement, the Tuskegee Health Benefit Plan was established to provide the lifetime health-care services (Centers for Disease Control and Prevention, 2011). In 1995, the program was expanded to include health and medical benefits. The infected wives, ex-wives, and widows received medical and health benefits. The last widow receiving benefits died on January 27, 2009. Currently, there are sixteen offspring who receive lifetime medical and health benefits (Centers for Disease Control and Prevention, 2011).

Further Implications: Medical Mistrust Among African-American Males

The Tuskegee Syphilis Study damaged the trust of African-Americans, especially African-American males, toward public health awareness and studies conducted by public health entities. The syphilis study reinforced African-Americans' distrust of the medical establishment, public-health programs, and vaccinations. As a significant result, many African-American males are hesitant to receive preventive care or participate in medical trials by public health officials and institutions (CNN, 2008).

Recommended Modifications to Informed Consent

The writer offers several modifications to informed consent that can modify how it is obtained and how practices related to informed consent may become more ethical.

• Animal experiments should be conducted before human experiments. The animal experiments can demonstrate whether treatment is ineffective or even dangerous, thus avoiding human experimentation. Animal experiments can also reveal side effects that may occur in human subjects (Standler, 1997).

• Only conduct new experiments. Researchers should conduct a thorough search of the medical and biological literature before conducting human experimentation. Research that has already been conducted should not be repeated unless there is a significant improvement in methodology or reason to suspect mistakes in the previous experiment (Standler, 1997).

• The study's benefit to society should outweigh the risks to the research subjects. These benefits should be analyzed by attorneys and the clergy in order to provide objectivity. The approval of an experimental protocol should be made by a review committee whose members have a voting majority of nonphysicians (Standler, 1997).

• Experiment on victims of disease and/or injury. Treatments should be tested on a group of people who could benefit from the medical treatment. An outside observer should observe the research subjects in the treatment group in order to measure the side effects of treatment and evidence of benefits. If the treatment group is experiencing serious side effects, the treatment should be discontinued early. If the treatment group has high benefits, then it is unethical to continue treatment while denying those benefits to the control group (Standler, 1997).

• Take care of subjects before the trial. Before the research is conducted, the researchers should disclose to the subjects any risks as a result of participation in the study (Standler, 1997).

- Research subjects should share in the rewards from developments due to their participation. They have a right to financial rewards generated by the studies in which they participate. Because their participation was essential, they should be paid for their time in addition to reimbursement of any expenses or loss of wages (Standler, 1997).

References

Berg, J. W.; Appelbaum, P. S.; Parker, L. S.; and Lidz, C. W. (2001). *Informed Consent: Legal Theory and Clinical Practice*. Oxford University Press.

Centers for Disease Control and Prevention (2011). *The Tuskegee Timeline*. Retrieved from http://www.cdc.gov/tuskegee/timeline.htm

Centers for Disease Control and Prevention (2011). *Research implications: How Tuskegee changed research practices*. Retrieved from http://www.cdc.gov/tuskegee/after.htm

CNN (2008). *Did Tuskegee damage trust on clinical trials?* Retrieved from http://cnn.com/2008?HEALTH03/17/clinical.trials.ap/index.html

Coy, J. A. (1989). "Autonomy-based informed consent: Ethical implications for patient noncompliance," *Physical Therapy, 69* (10), pg. 40–47.

Dunn, L. B.; Nowrangi, M. A.; Palmer, B. W.; Jeste, D. V.; and Saks, E. R. (2006, August). "Assessing decisional capacity for clinical research or treatment: A review of instruments," The *American Journal of Psychiatry, 163* (8), pg. 1323–1334.

Fisher, J. A. (2006). "Procedural misconceptions and informed consent: Insights from empirical research on the clinical trials industry," *Kennedy Institute of Ethics Journal, 16* (3), pg. 251–268.

Heintzelman, C. A. (2003). "The Tuskegee syphilis study and its implications for the twenty-first century," *The New Social Worker, 10* (4), pg. 1–5.

Office for Human Research Protections (2005). *Protection of Human Subjects. Title 45, Code of Federal Regulations, Part 46*. US Department of Health and Human Services.

Office for Human Research Protections (2008). Department of Health and Human Services. Retrieved from http://hhs.gov/ohrp/

Smith, S. (2010, October). "Wellesley professor unearths a horror: Syphilis experiments in Guatemala," *The Boston Globe*. Retrieved from http://www.bostonglobe.com

Solomon, R. C. (2006, August). "Ethical issues in medical malpractice," *Emergency Medical Clinics North American Journal*, 24 (3), pg. 733–47.

Standler, R. B. (1997). *Nonconsensual medical experiments on human beings*. Retrieved from http://www.rbs2.com/humres.htm

The Presidential Commission for the Study of Bioethical Issues. (2011). *Social justice and ethical issues: Transcript from March 1, 2011, in Washington, DC*. Retrieved from http://www.bioethics.gov/transcripts/human-subjects-protection/030111/social-justice-and-ethics-issues.html

The US National Archives and Records Administration. (2011). Tuskegee Patient Medical Files. Retrieved from http://www.archives.gov/southeast/finding-aids/tuskegee.html

Tuskegee University Manual for Institutional Review Board (2005). Retrieved on January 12, 2011 from www.tuskegee.edu

Informed Consent: Global Bioethical Perspectives of the Tuskegee and Guatemala Syphilis Studies

Obiora N. Anekwe

Abstract

The commonality among the Tuskegee Syphilis Study and the Guatemalan STD Study centered on the lack of informed consent among American government and medical researchers from the 1930s through the 1970s. The paper will explore cultural customs and language among these two different populations in the Americas and how such differences validate the need for cultural awareness among scientific researchers. The ethical concept of universalism will be highlighted in regard to the race and culture of African-American males in Macon County, Tuskegee, Alabama, and the male prisoners in Guatemala experimented upon in studies conducted by the United States Public Health Services.

Introduction

Universalism would contend that ethical principles remain the same, no matter where a medical research study is being conducted in the world. The paper will discuss the complexities of carrying modern research practices across cultural boundaries. It is both possible and necessary to stay true to ethical standards—such as informed consent—while also respecting the culture of those who are participating in a medical research study (Macklin 2011). Accordingly, "custom, culture, and tradition cannot provide a justification for departing from ethical principles" (Macklin 2011). The paper will additionally explore examples of this bioethical concept by highlighting two main studies that focused on the lack of informed consent among two vastly different cultural populations in the world. We will begin with a general definition of informed consent, which is a centerpiece of both studies due to the lack of its usage.

A Definition of Informed Consent

Informed consent usually refers to consent that a person gives that meets certain minimum standards. Further, an informed consent can be given based upon a clear understanding of the facts, implications, and future consequences of an action. In order to provide informed consent, the person involved in a study must have adequate reasoning faculties and be in possession of relevant facts at the time consent is given (Berg et al 2001). Impairments in reasoning and judgment such as basic intellectual/emotional immaturity, high levels of stress, severe mental illness, intoxication, severe sleep deprivation, Alzheimer's disease, or being in a coma constitute examples of impaired consent. The term *informed consent* was first used in the 1957 medical malpractice case by attorney Paul G. Gebhard (Solomon 2006).

The Tuskegee Syphilis Study: A Historical Background

In 1932, the Tuskegee Syphilis Study, properly known as the United States Public Health Study of Untreated Syphilis in the Negro Male (1932–1972), was a study by the United States government in which six hundred low income African-American males were recruited (399 of whom were infected with syphilis and 201 of whom were not). The men were recruited from Macon County, Alabama, and misled to believe that they were receiving free treatment for "bad blood," a euphemism for syphilis, which was epidemic in the county and surrounding areas (Word Press 2010). Throughout the forty-year study, treatment for syphilis was never provided to these men (Word Press 2010). Additionally, penicillin was withheld from the men once it was discovered that the drug could cure the disease and relieve the pain associated with the disease.

The Guatemala Syphilis Study: A Historical Background

Originally entitled, "Experimental Studies on Human Inoculation with Syphilis, Gonorrhea, and Chancroid," the Guatemala Syphilis Study was led by the efforts of American physician, Dr. John C. Cutler, one of the key physicians in the Tuskegee Syphilis Study. This paper focuses on experimentations involving syphilis in the Guatemalan prison system from 1947 to 1948.

In Guatemala, US clinical researchers intentionally exposed hundreds of people to syphilis, gonorrhea, and chancroid, only treating roughly half of those exposed (Cook 2011). In particular, the researchers conducted intentional exposure experiments involving syphilis with 688 subjects, including commercial sex workers, prisoners, and psychiatric patients (Presidential Commission for the Study of Bioethical Issues 2011). Within the prison population, a total of 219 prisoners were included in these clinical trials through exposure to infected commercial sex workers and/or artificial inoculations with infectious material (Presidential Commission for the Study of Bioethical Issues 2011).

Race and Culture of the Black Rural South: The Tuskegee Syphilis Study

Reverby notes that "as with other stories of critical importance in our national heritage, and especially those that focus on race and sexuality, the study endures on the cusp of memory and fact and in imagination, nightmare, and historical accounting at the same moment" (2011, 23). Cultural and regional differences, such as African-American southern dialect and social and class status, were systematically used as determinates in levels of intelligence, or the lack thereof, for minority populations in Tuskegee, Alabama.

The belief that African-Americans were sexually promiscuous was used to validate arguments that African-Americans were more likely to contract syphilis. This argument, along with the belief that the black male participants were educationally deprived, justified the blatant misinformation expressed to participants that they were being treated for "bad blood" rather than informing them that they had syphilis and treating them for the disease.

Some media outlets have simplified the description of the African-American men involved in the Tuskegee Syphilis Study as "399 Alabama black rural sharecropping illiterate men" without differentiating the occupational, educational, and personal identities of the men (Reverby 2001, 25). They became as a group, every southern black man, available as symbols of victimization and invisibility. The author of this paper would argue that the continuation of false representation in movies and books perpetuates victimization and exploitation of these deceased men and their family members.

Race and Culture of the Male Prison Population: The Guatemala Syphilis Study

Race was clearly a significant component of the Guatemalan experiments. At the time of the Study, many physicians believed that syphilis affected different races differently (Presidential Commission for the Study of Bioethical Issues 2011). Although Dr. Cutler did not discuss sexual promiscuity in his final reports, he does "partially account for the low gonorrhea transmission rate by the 'duration of coitus' in the 'culture group' involved in the Guatemalan army experiments" (Presidential Commission for the Study of Bioethical Issues 2011, 72–73).

Within prison populations in Guatemala, prison inmates were viewed as an isolated population that could be used for "normal exposure" to sexually transmitted diseases (i.e. sexual intercourse) (Presidential Commission for the Study of Bioethical Issues 2011). A large portion of the prison population consisted of indigenous Guatemalans, referred to by the US clinical doctors as "Indians" (Presidential Commission for the Study of Bioethical Issues 2011). Despite the pervasive belief that the effects of syphilis varied among races, Dr. Cutler's final Syphilis Report concluded that the researchers found no evidence of racial immunity in the Guatemalan research subjects experimented upon (Presidential Commission for the Study of Bioethical Issues 2011).

Universalism in Light of Both Studies

Universalism holds that ethics applies universally, that is for "all similarly situated individuals" regardless of culture, race, sex, religion, nationality, sexuality, or any other distinguishing feature (Philosophical Dictionary 2011). In both studies presented, ethical universalism was excluded because the clinical researchers, who worked for the United States Public Health Services in both cases, believed that the universal ethical principles did not apply to the vulnerable populations experimented upon due to their race, sex, and nationality. Although a revised and more formalized concept of informed consent was not developed until after the conclusion of the Tuskegee and Guatemalan Studies, the various aspects of informed consent were formulated from the unethical and even, as some scholars contend, immoral medical practices of these and similar studies nationally and internationally. In reflection, universal ethical concepts such as informed consent were not applied to vulnerable populations such as minorities, the mentally and physically challenges, and children until federal laws, provisions, policies, and governmental agencies were established to protect such populations.

Because the researchers worked for the United States government, their beliefs were further reinforced by the state and federal laws regarding racial segregation in North America, expressed beliefs of human equality and dignity of racial and ethnic minorities in North and Central America, and governmental and state laws which prohibited the civil rights of racial and ethnic minorities in North America until the 1960s. In emphasizing the fact that racial minorities were not considered worthy of dignity in the medical setting by white public health officials and even African-American officials, it would be easy to see why universalism was nonexistent in the ethical belief system of the clinical researchers who conducted the studies. Rather than viewing the men who participated in these studies as men with equal rights who deserved full informed consent, many governmental clinical researchers viewed the men as a means to an end, with no human value, dignity, or rights. Clearly, the negative physical and mental repercussions for the males participating in the two studies outweighed any benefits from participating in the studies.

Concluding Remarks

The ethical responses to the Tuskegee and Guatemala Syphilis Studies demonstrate the lack of humane and ethical experimentation practices that occurred among vulnerable populations based on race, class, and health-care disparities before the 1970s. Consequentially, the dominant lesson that emerges from these two nonconsensual clinical experimentations and its efforts to eliminate race-based medical practice centers on a continued effort to emphasize the constitutive nature of human equality, the need for full disclosure, and informed consent. As future Bioethicists, it is our duty to shed light on the unethical medical and health-care practices of the past in order to correct them for future generations and ensure that they do not occur again.

References

Berg, J. W., Appelbaum, P. S., Parker, L. S., and Lidz, C. W. 2001. *Informed consent: legal theory and clinical practice.* Oxford University Press.

Macklin, R. 2011. *Expert advocates ethical constancy in research.* Retrieved from http://www.fordham.edu/Campus_Resources/eNewsroom/topstories

Philosophical Dictionary 2011. Retrieved from http://www.philosophypages.com/dy/u.htm

Presidential Commission for the Study of Bioethical Issues September 2011. "'Ethically impossible': STD research in Guatemala from 1946 to 1948." Retrieved from www.bioethics.gov

Reverby, S. M. 2001. More than fact and fiction: Cultural memory and the Tuskegee Syphilis Study. *The Hastings Center Report,* 31 (5): 22–28.

Reverby, S. M. 2010. "After the media frenzy, preventing another 'Guatemala,'" Retrieved from http://www.thehastingscenter.org/Post.aspx?id=4919

Solomon, R. C., August 2006. "Ethical issues in medical malpractice," *Emergency MedicalClinics North American Journal,* 24 (3), pg. 733–747.

Word Press 2010. "Keep the ethical light burning." Retrieved from http://keeptheethicallightburning.org/tuskegee-case/

Physicians' Responsibilities and Patients' Rights
Obiora N. Anekwe

The rights of patients have not always been dominant in health care and medicine. Historically and philosophically, patients were not always viewed as equal parties in the decision-making process; rather the doctor was symbolically viewed as the sole arbiter of medical decision-making. The four models of the physician-patient relationship will be explored in this essay. This paper will discuss the opposing perspective that the four models that exist are not sufficient for effective physician-patient relationships and question whether an alternative model is necessary. Lastly, the writer will identify one model from the course readings that is most effective, which preserves patients' rights and physicians' responsibilities, and/or present an alternative model that is more transparent in nature.

According to Emanuel and Emanuel (1992), four models of the physician-patient relationship exist. These models are the paternalistic, informative, interpretive, and deliberative. Each particular model is unique and reflective of philosophical perspectives that compliment the physician-patient relationship. The first model, known as the paternalistic model, is authoritative and parental in that the doctor serves as the expert who determines the most effective means of treatment with the patient's consent (Emanuel and Emanuel, 1992). But an underlying limitation of such a model is that the physician does not necessarily take into account pertinent medical opinions or input by the patient who is being treated (Emanuel and Emanuel, 1992). Consequentially, this model runs the risk of providing ineffective medical care due to a lack of insight from the patient.

The second model Emanuel and Emanuel cite is the informative model. In this model, information is provided from the physician based solely on scientific or medical data, including the risks and benefits of possible treatments (Emanuel and Emanuel,

1992). Ultimately, the patient is left to make the best decision of medical care or treatment based on the information provided (Emanuel and Emanuel, 1992). Although the informative model empowers the patient to make the final medical decision, it disallows critical medical opinions by the physician that may impact the outcome of medical treatment.

The third model, commonly referred to as the interpretive model, is perhaps one of the most effective in the physician-patient relationship. Similar to the informative model, this model not only provides medical data for the patient in order to help him or her decide the best means of medical treatment, it also empowers the physician to interpret the medical data and to provide options for the patient (Emanuel and Emanuel, 1992). One role that physicians possess in the interpretive model is that of counselor, which requires skills in listening and explaining.

The fourth model, the deliberative model, is the most assertive model of the physician-patient relationship. The physician and the patient are both actively involved in formulating alternative options for medical treatment. Moral persuasion is a unique attribute of this model in that the patient's health-related values are discussed with the doctor, which ultimately assists the patient in deciding what type of treatment is most suitable (Emanuel and Emanuel, 1992).

Emanuel and Emanuel stress that a fifth model of the physician-patient relationship can be added, the instrumental model. Within this model, the patient's values are not significant; rather the central goal of treatment or lack thereof is altruistic in nature, such as the good of society or progression of scientific discovery. At this point within the paper, the writer would like to further explore the nature of the instrumental model and its correlation to the Tuskegee Syphilis Study.

One of the most unethical clinical trials that dramatically changed the dynamics of the physician-patient relationship was the Tuskegee Syphilis Study, held from 1932 to 1972 in Macon County, Alabama, and surrounding counties. The Tuskegee Syphilis Study had its origins in race-based medicine rooted in the early eugenics movement. Public health doctors involved in the Tuskegee Syphilis Study convinced the male subjects involved in the study that they were being treated for their "bad blood" (syphilis), although they were not. A type of deadly deception essentially took place where many African-American men involved in the experiment eventually died as a result of nontreatment for syphilis, even when penicillin became widely available for treatment of the disease in the 1940s.

As depicted in Display Image 1, doctors involved in the syphilis study functioned within the instrumental model. They were the experts who medically directed the study participants, updated the weight and physical condition of the male participants, and regularly tested the blood to check the syphilis status of participants who were in the nonsyphilitic group. Throughout the forty-year span of the study, the participants were never provided medical information as to why painful tests such as spinal taps were conducted without anesthesia, which eventually caused physical harm and even eventual death for some male subjects.

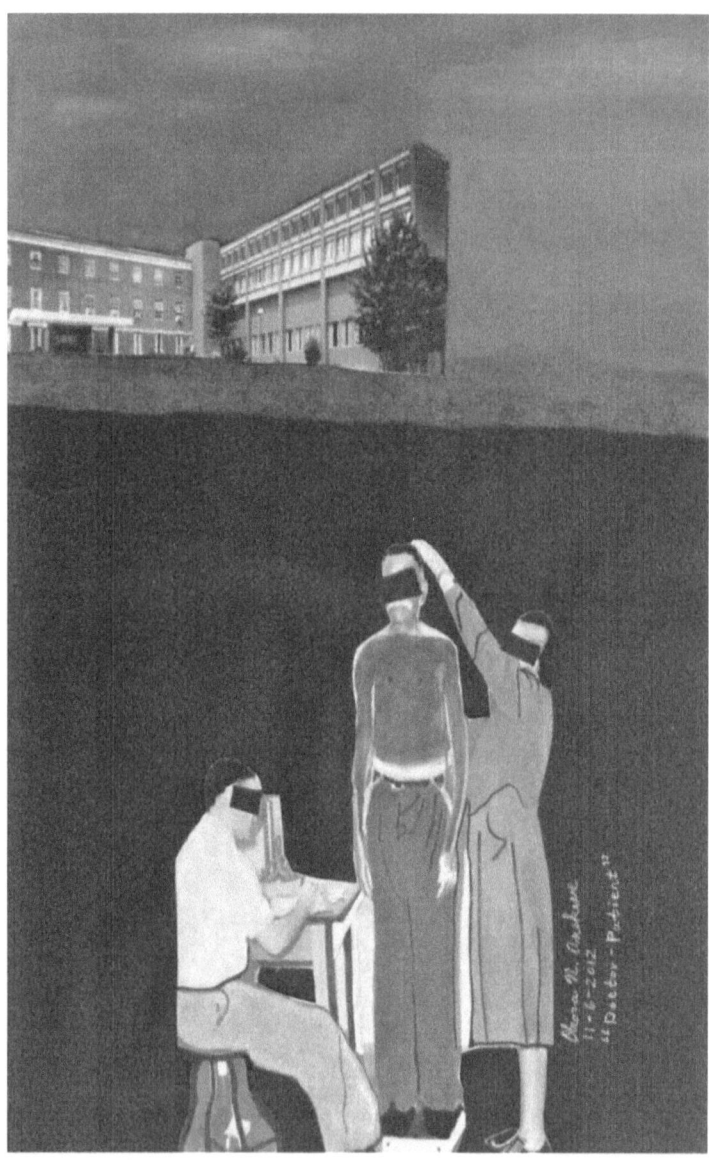

Doctor-Patient, by Obiora N. Anekwe. The art collage shows a public health doctor and nurse checking the height and weight of a male participant in the Tuskegee Syphilis Study. The upper left hand corner of the collage shows the John A. Andrew Memorial Hospital on the campus of Tuskegee Institute (now Tuskegee University), where the Tuskegee Syphilis Study was conducted.

The public health doctors who conducted the Tuskegee Syphilis Study defended their medical actions of deception and withholding of penicillin to treat the clinical trial participants based on a utilitarian approach to treatment, which emphasizes actions that promote the greater good of society. For example, although penicillin was available for syphilis treatment in the 1940s during the study, participants were prevented from treatment because doctors wanted to measure the progress of untreated syphilis in the African-American male body. Their justification for nontreatment was systematically based on a belief that if the nontreatment could be observed, then medical doctors could prove that the black male body reacted to a sexually transmitted disease differently than the white male body. To the public health physicians, these observations were more important than the treatment of syphilis. This form of race-based medical practice was not uncommon in clinical trials in the early 1900s due to the advent of bad eugenics, which was also based on the belief that the sacrifice of a few would ultimately benefit scientific inquiry and the greater society.

To the contrary, one could also emphasize a more empathetic approach to the physician-patient relationship as it relates to the Tuskegee Syphilis Study and utilitarianism. Even though medical practice concerns the betterment of society, it can also be inclusive of the fact that treating people well during treatment decreases the likelihood of the kind of negative backlash that once plagued unethical clinical trials, such as the Tuskegee Syphilis Study. Although the medical outcome is for the greater societal good, empathetic treatment may also need to be employed in order to prevent public outcry or unease, which may decrease the likelihood that people would want to participate in future clinical trials. One could additionally argue that if a more caring approach to medical treatment existed, such as providing penicillin to syphilitic participants, the African-American community would not be as hesitant to participate in clinical trials today.

In order to build a more effective physician-patient model, one must reject the idea that the end justifies the means and embrace the notion that the means used in past medical endeavors need to be reevaluated in order to create a better process and outcome with greater results? From a consequentialist perspective, one would argue that the Tuskegee Syphilis Study, based upon the instrumental belief that doctors should instruct patients without regard to the patients' values, was justified because the medical contributions of study participants brought greater insight into how the black male body reacted to syphilis, even if many men involved in the study died as a *consequence* of nontreatment of syphilis. In this case, the consequentialist would contend that the end clearly justified the means, even if such means involved medical deception and even death for patients who did not receive penicillin even when it was made available in the 1940s.

But another school of philosophical thought, known as *deontology*, would argue that no matter the medical outcome, what occurred during the 40-year period of the Tuskegee Syphilis Study was unjustifiably unethical and no outcome could justify its disrespect for universal human rights and dignity. The deontologist would contend that medical deception and the withholding of valuable treatment for patients in need of treatment was then and is now intrinsically wrong and fundamentally unethical. Therefore, the end is not justified if the means are unethical in nature and scope. It can reasonably be argued that a more effective and inclusive physician-patient relationship model should be introduced that decreases the likelihood of unjustified mistreatment of patients.

One can clearly observe that due to the consequentialist approach to the Tuskegee Syphilis Study and other similar unethical clinical trials, this inclusive model, known as the *informed consent-decision-making model* (IC-DM Model), provides a more effective physician-patient relationship model than the models presented earlier by Emanuel and Emanuel (1992). The IC-DM model, a hybrid of the four primary models, is based on formalized and purposeful informed consent that promotes a medical culture in which both the doctor and the patient make medical decisions based upon medical benefits and needs of the patient. The ethical elements of respect for patients and dignity of patient rights are attributes that both the patient and doctor share. If such a model existed during the occurrence of the syphilis study, many detrimental and unethical aspects of the study may not have occurred.

Emanuel and Emanuel (1992) provided four models for the physician-patient medical relationship. These models provided structured frameworks for how doctors and patients interact in a medical relationship, but each model seemed to lack a comprehensive view of how such relationships should be conducted with the patient's best interest in mind. The instrumental model, which was not explored as deeply by Emanuel and Emanuel (1992), focused on the physician's authoritative direction without any insight or consent from the patient. As a result, such clinical trials as the Tuskegee Syphilis Study were conducted without the patient's informed consent. But the writer suggests that a more patient-centered model exists that takes into consideration the patient's right to have formalized and informed consent due to the unethical practices in some previous clinical trials. The IC-DM Model provides an enhanced view that patients have medical rights and they can refuse treatment or participation in clinical trials if they so desire. Based on mutual collaborative medical outcomes, this model provides an ethical framework consistent with universal human rights and the dignity of human existence. Therefore, such a model is bound to be an effective example to both physicians and patients in how to interact with one another for the patient's common good.

References

Childress, J. F. and Siegler, M. (1984). "Metaphors and models of doctor-patient relationships." *Theoretical Medicine, 5*, 17–34.

Emanuel, E. J. and Emanuel, L. L. (1992, April 22/29). "Four models of the physician-patient relationship." *Journal of the American Medical Association, 267* (16), 2221–26.

The National Archives and Records Administration (2012). Southeast Region, Morrow, Georgia.

The Tuskegee University Archives (2011). Tuskegee, Alabama.

Philosophical and Practical Considerations for Just and Equitable Health Care in America
Obiora N. Anekwe

We must not see any person as an abstraction. Instead, we must see in every person a universe with its own secrets, with its own treasures, with its own sources of anguish, and with some measure of triumph.
Elie Wiesel
from The Nazi Doctors and the Nuremberg Code

Introductory Statement

Jesus the Christ once proclaimed that "the poor you will always have with you" (Matthew 26:11). His acknowledgment is evidence that the needy and disenfranchised are among us even in today's society. They are affected by limited access to health care that eventually affects society as a whole. Public policy, public voices, and action coalitions have attempted to close the gap between those who have health care and those who do not. But how can practical solutions to health-care disparities resolve this contemporary issue?

Philosophical thinkers like John Locke and John Rawls have hinted at solutions to health-care inequality in writings centered on justice and fairness, even to the extent of reparations for victims. Studies such as the Tuskegee Syphilis Study and the Henrietta Lacks Experiment serve as examples in how inequity in health care promoted and legitimized unethical treatments of vulnerable populations in clinical trials. Do such populations deserve reparations for crimes committed against them by public health-care physicians? Should these same officials be criminally and ethically accountable for their unethical and immoral medical actions against vulnerable populations? Modern philosopher John Rawls further explores the theory of justice as fairness that can also be applied to issues of inequality and inequity in health care.

Many libertarian opponents would disagree and argue that what is merely unfortunate is not unfair. Through the libertarian perspective, society has no obligation to provide the poor with what they are missing. In this essay, I will explore both sides of the issue of inequity and inequality in health care under the philosophical idea that they curtail national growth and prosperity. I plan to argue that if we, as a citizenry, cannot provide health-care resources and access to our greatest in need, then we, as an American people, cannot succeed as we should.

The Tuskegee Syphilis Study: A Brief Background

From 1932 to 1972, the longest clinical trial in the history of North America took place in Macon County in the southern city of Tuskegee Institute, Alabama. For the purpose of the paper, I shall refer to this clinical trial as the *Tuskegee Syphilis Study*. The syphilis study was housed at the Tuskegee Institute (now Tuskegee University) in the campus clinical facility of the John A. Andrew Memorial Hospital. Officially it was known as the US Public Health Service Syphilis Study at Tuskegee, and under it the US Public Health Service staff recruited hundreds of African-American men in rural Alabama in order to study and clinically measure the effects of syphilis in the black male body. "Early in the study, 399 men with late latent syphilis, and 201 men without syphilis were initially enrolled. As the study evolved, additional participants were added, so the number of men in the study varies according to the source" (Centers for Disease Control and Prevention, 2012, p. 1). At present, all the African-American men who were study participants are deceased, but many of their family members live on.

In order to test the doctors' scientific hypothesis that the African-American male body would react differently to syphilis than the white male body, public health doctors did not treat the men for syphilis but deceived them in order to measure the validity of their hypothesis. Even after penicillin was discovered in the 1940s, treatment was still withheld from the men in order to measure the effects of syphilis until death. A number of local African-American and white physicians were involved in the practice of withholding treatment for syphilis (Centers for Disease Control and Prevention, 2012). Additionally, a number of Tuskegee Institute faculty and staff were paid by the Public Health Service in order to formally serve as human subject recruiters, researchers, and medical personnel for the study (Centers for Disease Control and Prevention, 2012). Many of the men died from the effects of the disease. The medical practices were not scientific but influenced by racial stereotypes about the black male body that have been promoted since the days of slavery in the Americas.

The Henrietta Lacks Experiment (The HeLa Experiment): A Brief Background

Henrietta Lacks was a poor black tobacco farmer whose cells were taken without her consent in 1951 (Skloot, 2010). This population of cells, known as HeLa cells, became one of the most significant tools in medicine used to develop the polio vaccine, cloning, gene mapping, and in vitro fertilization (IVF) (Skloot,

2010). Although Mrs. Lacks never received any compensation for the usage of her unique cells in human research, these cells have been bought and sold by the billions. The name of the cells, *HeLa* (pronounced hee-lah) is derived from the first two letters of Mrs. Henrietta Lacks first and last name (Skloot, 2010).

Mrs. Lacks's primary physician referred her to The Johns Hopkins Hospital, an affiliate of The Johns Hopkins University, in order to examine a lump in her cervix, which was later discovered to be cancerous. Johns Hopkins was the hospital of choice due to the fact that it was the only hospital in the area that would treat black patients. Nevertheless, Mrs. Lacks was still medically treated in the "colored" section of the hospital due to segregation. During her radiation treatments for the tumor, two samples of Mrs. Lacks's cervix were removed (a healthy part and a cancerous part) without her permission. These cells were eventually given to Dr. George Otto Gey in other to multiply them and conduct biomedical research. Known for their unique ability to multiply and replicate quickly, these cells are now commonly used in biomedical research. For the purposes of this paper, I will refer to the unethical extraction of Henrietta Lacks's cells and the subsequent usage of them in biomedical research as the *Henrietta Lacks Experiment*.

John Rawls's Theory of Justice as Fairness

John Rawls is perhaps one of the most well-known theorists on the philosophical concept of justice and fairness. A just and equitable health-care system preserves the right and ability of people to participate in the social, political and economic life of society (Daniels, 2012). Rawls's theory of justice as fairness assumes that we have a completely healthy society. He argued that, "a just society must assure people equal basic liberties, guarantee that the right of political participation has roughly equal value for all, provide a robust form of equal opportunity, and limit inequalities to those that benefit the least advantaged" (Daniels, 2012, p. 11). He concludes that once these requirements of justice are met, we, as a society, can be assured that respect for self-worth is visible and evident. The fair terms of cooperation identified through these principles eventually promote our political and social well-being (Daniels, 2012). In essence, if the least among us are provided with equal social necessities, such as health care, our general population benefits politically and socially because society, as a whole, is better off with a healthy and robust body of people.

The basic tenants of Rawls's theory of justice as fairness (equal liberties, equal opportunity, a fair distribution of resources, and acknowledgement of our self-respect) all contribute to the elimination of injustices in health care (Daniels, 2012). Therefore, social justice is inextricably connected to justice as a means to fairness in medicine and health care. The equal and fair distribution of health-care resources sustains all people as full and engaged citizens. Equitable health care also maintains the normal functioning of individuals, protecting a person's fair share of opportunities to succeed (Daniels, 2012). In other words, people make better and more informed decisions and choices when they are healthy.

Rawls's theory "assures people of equal basic liberties, including equal access to political participation; guarantees a robust form of equal opportunity; and imposes significant constraints on inequalities" (Daniels, Kennedy, and Kawachi, 1999, p. 217). Democratic equality is the central outcome. It ensures that all citizens have the social bases of self-respect with the conviction that prospects in life are fair (Daniels, Kennedy, and Kawachi, 1999). The concept of justice as fairness is unique to the discussion at hand because it explicitly supports a belief that equal opportunity (providing opportunity to those who have the least choices) could be extended to health care. Health care, in and of itself, is morally and ethically important in our discussion about inequity and inequality because it helps to preserve our status as fully functioning citizens. Just as equality in educational opportunity is significant to justice, so is equality in health care. Both go hand in hand in assuring a more perfect union.

In many ways, our health is affected by our social position or status and the underlying inequalities in our society (Daniels, 2012). Who we are in relation to our socioeconomic background, race, ethnicity, regional location, and gender are just a few factors that affect fairness and justice in health care. These social determinants clearly exist and are observed in immoral, unfair, unjust, and unethical medical practices such as those of the Tuskegee Syphilis Study and the Henrietta Lacks Experiment. In order to formulate a more robustly fair health-care system, void of blatant discriminatory practices, we must consider social justice measures that prevent unethical research and clinical measures.

The philosophical theory of justice as fairness serves as an effective model that can reduce the number of unethical health-care injustices perpetrated upon vulnerable populations. One explainable reason why human subjects involved in the Tuskegee Syphilis Study and the Henrietta Lacks's Experiment were selected and medically exploited was because both populations lacked access to equalized health-care resources in their respective communities. The African-American men involved in the syphilis study were primarily interested in participating in the clinical trial because doctors assured them that they would be treated free of charge for their "bad blood," a term used in their local community to describe people infected with syphilis.

As shown in Display Image 1, flyers were disseminated throughout the local community in order to recruit men to be a part of the study, promising that they would be treated for their "bad blood," although they were not. Due to public segregation of hospitals in the 1930s, when the syphilis study was first initiated, the closest and most accessible hospital for nonmilitary males was the John A. Andrew Memorial Hospital, founded on the campus of Tuskegee Institute by African-Americans to medically treat all patients in the local Tuskegee-Macon County community.

If health-care education resource inequalities and segregation of hospital services were not prevalent during the occurrence of the Tuskegee Syphilis Study, many African-American men might not have participated in this clinical trial, because they would have sought out or been provided equalized health education and medical care for syphilis.

Henrietta Lacks sought out medical care for her illness in the 1950s at one of the best medical facilities in the country, The Johns Hopkins Hospital in Baltimore, Maryland. But medical facilities and resources at the hospital were still segregated. As a black woman who was not provided proper consent about the full extent of her medical treatment and extraction of her unique cells, doctors at The Johns Hopkins Hospital exploited her due to her lack of educational and health-care resources.

As a result, her cells, known as HeLa cells, have been multiplied in the trillions in order to aid in experiments that have resulted in the cure for polio and research on cancer, just to name a few. Neither Mrs. Lacks nor her family were compensated for the extraction of her unique cells that have, ironically, made billions of dollars for research companies and saved the lives of millions of people through innovative research. Even today, some of her family members suffer from multiple illnesses and still lack fair and affordable health-care insurance, although their ancestor contributed so much to medical discoveries.

John Locke's Philosophical Emphasis on Human Liberty, Reparations, and Retributions

In order to move forward in our discussion of John Locke's philosophical emphasis on reparations and retributions, it would be practical to explain a basic attribute of his theory: retribution.

Retribution is the balancing of a wrong through punishment (Pollock, 2005). It is impersonal and balanced (Pollock, 2005). In a social contract, the state or governing institution has the right to inflict retribution or punishment upon guilty parties or criminals who transgress the individual rights of others. This concept is as ancient as Greek philosophy, which is also evident in the writings of Thomas Hobbs (*Leviathan*, 1651), Jean-Jacques Rousseau (*Du contrat social*, 1762), and the philosopher of focus in this essay, John Locke (*Two Treatises on Government*, 1690).

In Locke's *Two Treatises on Government* (1690), he acknowledges that all *men* are created equal in a state of nature by God. Thomas Jefferson, an American founding father, adopted this belief and incorporated it into the US Declaration of Independence. Such a belief holds that by naturalistic right, each person possesses the right to life, liberty, and the pursuit of happiness (or more directly, property). Therefore, those who infringe upon the rights of others should be held accountable to society.

As we observe the blatant disregard for patient rights as demonstrated in the Tuskegee Syphilis Study and the Henrietta Lacks Experiment, we see how individual rights to life and liberty were violated and disregarded. The purposeful failure to obtain informed consent from patients goes against the medical ideal of doing no harm. It is the duty of doctors to work in the best interests of patients rather than to work against every moral or ethical standard that exists in medical practice. Locke would clearly argue that both experiments violated these rights and, therefore, reparations need to be made in order to compensate individuals for their suffering.

But utilitarians would argue that Locke and Jefferson's writings never explicitly defined who men are. In other words, the definition of men with natural rights included white males but excluded enslaved blacks and women so that they did not possess these same rights in society during the time when Locke's *Two*

Treatises on Government (1690) or the Declaration of Independence were written. On that basis, the usefulness of an argument that contends that African-Americans involved in the two unethical experiments deserve retribution and compensation is without merit. As the utilitarian would state, what truly matters is that the larger society benefited from the usage of Mrs. Lacks's HeLa cells in order to discover medical cures. In addition, our greater society also benefited scientifically from knowing that the black male body does not react to syphilis any differently than the white male body.

In Chapter II (Sections 8 and 11) of *Two Treatises on Government*, Locke (1690) advocates for the punishment of crimes committed against society that violate the rights of others. He also indicates that reparations are viable options that may help restore violated liberties to victims, restrain others from committing unlawful acts in society. One could justifiably extend Locke's concept of reparations to include unethical and immoral transgressions against individuals in society who have been systematically stripped of their ethical and moral rights to proper and informed medical care. Therefore, reparations for victims or family members affected by these two unethical experiments are warranted. Reparations in both cases would help repair and mend past wrongs, dissuade others from conducting such unethical acts, and help heal the physical, mental, and spiritual wounds of the past.

Other ethicists who hold a utilitarian perspective would counter this argument and question the merit of reparations to victims when compensation, in and of itself, cannot wipe away past misdeeds. They would contend that what's done is done, and no form of compensation can make up for past indiscretions. Therefore, we simply should learn from previous unethical experiments in order to positively impact future generations in society. Medical contributions from both experiments far outweighed any wrongful acts that were committed against individual victims. So the end justified the means. Lastly, the vulnerable populations involved in both types of experiments clearly suffered from diseases that they probably would have died from anyway without treatment; therefore, the sacrifice of their lives was worth their contributions to medicine and the greater good.

The Utilitarian Perspective of Justice, Fairness, and Retribution

Many libertarians argue that it is impossible for the state to give victims of injustice what they positively deserve. Under a utilitarian approach, what is good is that which benefits the many (Pollock, 2005). Therefore, even if an unjust, immoral, or unethical act was painful to an individual, if the majority in society benefited, then such an act is defined as good. According to their philosophical approach, medical harm caused by the lack of informed consent in patients involved in the Tuskegee Syphilis Study and the Henrietta Lacks Experiment may have been unethical and unjust, but if medical discoveries benefited the greater society, then such unethical actions are considered good.

Some public health medical doctors involved in the syphilis study have publicly defended the premise of their experimental work by contending that they now know for a fact that the African-American male body physically reacts to syphilis in the same way as the white male body, especially during the latent stage of the disease. Other scholars would argue that such a defense still does not ethically justify medical deception and uninformed consent, which caused the deaths of hundreds of African-American men who were not treated for syphilis.

As shown in Display Image 2, the artwork titled *Human Subjects* illustrates how African-American male participants involved in the Tuskegee Syphilis Study were photographed with their shirts off and with their faces shown, as evident in the original archival photograph. As the artist, I abstractly blackened the faces of the men in order to protect their identities and to further emphasize their physical attributes such as bodily strength, which inadvertently helped to promote the unfounded medical stereotype that the African-American male body was more physically resistant to syphilis than the white male body.

Further Utilitarian Arguments

Utilitarian critics of retributions and reparations for unethical deeds committed against minority populations would first argue that the state is a collective body that is imperfect; thus it cannot be fair in its own allocation of justice and equality. Secondly, the utilitarian would contend that compensation for a violation of another's right could not realistically restore the moral balance. Even after the moral or ethical offender compensates the victim for a harm done, he or she is still morally and ethically deficient (Gaus, 1999). Furthermore, even after all possible compensation has been provided, the utilitarian would argue that the harm could not be undone. The wrong still remains.

Thirdly, the utilitarian would question how one would define a *victim* of an unethical medical act. What criteria can one use to access victimhood when crimes against people are not equal to one another? The utilitarian approach would be skeptical of how the word *victim* is defined and contend that some people in society could describe themselves as victims when, in actuality, they are not. Therefore, there is a great possibility that some in society could take advantage of the state and define themselves as victims only with the intent of receiving compensation. Fourthly, utilitarian critics would question how society would define parties who inflict wrongs on others as *criminals*. Although an action against a person or segment of a population can be unethical, immoral, or even unjust, there may not exist laws that could enable the government to charge wrongdoers for such actions and prosecute them as criminals. And lastly, utilitarians would argue that just because an immoral or unethical act was committed against a person or group of people does not necessarily mean that it was a crime according to the laws and bylaws of society. Therefore, the state is not under any obligation to compensate or provide punishment for such acts.

Personal Perspectives

I feel a deep connection to what occurred in the Tuskegee Syphilis Study and the Henrietta Lacks Experiment because I was born in 1974 on the campus of Tuskegee Institute (now Tuskegee University) at the John A. Andrew Memorial Hospital in Tuskegee Institute, Alabama, where the syphilis study was conducted. My father, Gregory E. Anekwe, PhD, worked as a biochemist and associate professor of biochemistry at the George Washington Carver Research Foundation. The HeLa Cell Program began at the George Washington Carver Research Foundation on the campus of Tuskegee Institute. My brother, Ejinkonye C. Anekwe, PhD, performed cytogenetics research involving HeLa cells.

It was not until I conducted my own independent research about both the Tuskegee Syphilis Study and the Henrietta Lacks Experiment that I fully understood the ramifications of both studies in biomedical research. I have had the unique opportunity to interview and know many family members of men involved in the Tuskegee Syphilis Study. Additionally, I have spoken with some family members of Mrs. Lacks. In 2012, the Lacks family visited the Legacy Museum at Tuskegee University during the opening of a joint exhibition about the Tuskegee Syphilis Study and the Henrietta Lacks Experiment.

A More Philosophically Balance Approach: Tangible Solutions to Equitable and Just Reparations

At this point in the paper, I would like to provide a more philosophically balanced approach to justice, equity, and equality to health care. My approach rests on the foundation of holistic healing for both the victim and initiator of injustice. For our purposes, my philosophical concept shall be described as Social Equality through Holistic Healing (SE-HH). This concept is inclusive of elements such as public apologies, monetary compensation, accessible health care and education, humanistic documentary interviewing, and art as a means to healing. It also contends that both parties, the victim and initiator of injustices and inequalities in health care, need radical healing: spiritually, physically, mentally, and emotionally. Both parties have to acknowledge the wrongfulness of the unethical and immoral medical act that occurred. But most importantly, tangible solutions should be initiated in order to foster an environment of healing and radical change in how human subjects are treated in medical research.

My Social Equality through Holistic Healing Approach is rooted in the basic societal tenants of West African cultures that render justice through holistic measures. Both the victim and instigator of unethical acts against society actively participate in the healing or restoration process. It is an alternative to mere strict punishment of guilty parties. Rather, it seeks to bring healing or wholeness through direct and tangible measures that benefit the victims and/or family members affected by unethical medical crimes. Tangible solutions involve both the perpetrator and the victim of a medical wrongdoing initiated by federal and state governments, medical bodies, and/or educational institutions.

Because of my personal and family connection to the two unethical experiments, I would like to provide five tangible means of holistic healing for family members of victims affected by both the Tuskegee Syphilis Study and the Henrietta Lacks Experiment. Family members who were affected by these experiments are highlighted in these healing recommendations because there are no known living survivors from among the subjects of these experiments. Therefore, it would make logical sense that the descendants of these victims benefit from recommended policies and initiatives, which has not been the case so far. Nevertheless, these tangible healing initiatives include the following:

1) A public apology and acknowledgement should be given to the families of victims affected by the Tuskegee Syphilis Study and the Henrietta Lacks Experiment from the institutions directly involved in conducting these unethical clinical research experiments on their ancestors. These are the Tuskegee Institute (the John A. Andrew Memorial Hospital in Tuskegee, Alabama) and The Johns Hopkins University (The Johns Hopkins Hospital in Baltimore, Maryland). To date, there has not been a public apology from either institution for their role and involvement in serving as the research sites for two of the most unethical medical experiments in American history. A public apology by these institutions would serve as a starting point for healing for both the wrongdoers and the family members of victims. Although former President Clinton provided a formal apology in 1997 to victims of the Tuskegee Syphilis Study for the federal government's role in the syphilis study, the institution that housed the clinical trial for forty years has not apologized for their involvement.

2) A federally mandated act needs to be recommended in order to create a fund that will provide monetary compensation and free lifetime health care to family members affected by the Tuskegee Syphilis Study and the Henrietta Lacks Experiment. Family members of victims from the Tuskegee Syphilis Study have indicated to me through personal communication that they have yet to be properly compensated monetarily for the negative effects of the study. Victims of the syphilis study were provided monetary compensation as a result of a lawsuit settlement, but the money provided to these victims was such a minimum amount that it did not transfer from one generation to another. An out-of-court settlement

of ten million dollars was reached in 1974 with the parties. Each surviving subject was to be paid $37,500, each heir or representative of a diseased subject received fifteen thousand dollars, each member of the control group received sixteen thousand dollars, and the heir or a representative of each control subject received five thousand dollars (Centers for Disease Control and Prevention, 2012). These amounts are quite minimal compared to the physical, mental, and spiritual anguish many victims experienced as a result of participating in such an unjust and unethical study.

After former President Clinton publicly apologized in 1997 for the government's role in conducting the Tuskegee Syphilis Study, the Tuskegee Health Benefit Program (THBP) was established in order to provide comprehensive lifetime medical and health benefits to the affected widows and offspring of study participants. Currently, there are thirteen children and two grandchildren receiving medical and health benefits (Centers for Disease Control and Prevention, 2012). But I would contend that the program is not comprehensive enough, because there are many more relatives of victims who have not received free lifetime health-care services. In terms of the family members of Mrs. Henrietta Lacks, they have yet to be compensated monetarily for their ancestor's uninformed medical participation in the extraction of her cells, which have monetarily benefited a number of medical researchers, medical corporations, and research institutions. As indicated in a number of national interviews with family members of Mrs. Lacks, many of her descendants do not have health insurance and still lack proper health-care resources. Free lifetime health-care resources for family members of victims of both experiments would help decrease health-care disparities among these families and compensate for the medical deception doctors inflicted on their loved ones due to the lack of health-care resources and education.

3) A scholarship fund should be established for family members of the victims involved in the Tuskegee Syphilis Study and the Henrietta Lacks Experiment in order for them to attend college at Tuskegee University and The Johns Hopkins University, respectively. The Tuskegee Syphilis Study was conducted on the campus of Tuskegee Institute. Henrietta Lacks's unique cells were extracted from her body without her consent at The Johns Hopkins Hospital. Both educational institutions played a significant role in the perpetuation of unethical experiments conducted in American medicine. Therefore, these institutions must be held accountable for their misdeeds. Education provides a means by which acts of wrongfulness can be taught in order to prevent them from occurring again.

Tuskegee University and The Johns Hopkins University can play a lasting role in educating descendants of victims from the Tuskegee Syphilis Study and the Henrietta Lacks Experiment, respectively. Rather than creating wounds of despair, both institutions can serve as ladders of healing in order to decrease educational disparities. Research has indicated that many health-care disparities are connected to educational disparities as well. They go hand in hand. Therefore, prominent educational institutions can further educate descendants of former human subjects in order to create a sensible and safe environment of healing.

Although Rebecca Skloot, author of the book, *The Immortal Life of Henrietta Lacks*, established a foundation in order to provide college tuition assistance to family members affected by the Henrietta Lacks Experiment, a scholarship fund established by Tuskegee University and The Johns Hopkins

University would provide an active program of reconciliation and healing by these prominent institutions.

4) I, the writer, plan to produce and direct an educational documentary film, interviewing family members of victims affected by the Tuskegee Syphilis Study. Titled, *Ancestral Voices: A Documentary*, the film will provide primary accounts from family members who personally knew the men who were experimented upon in the syphilis study. This documentary will be the first visual project that only interviews family members affected by the syphilis study.

By making such a film, I intend for the general public to be able to understand the Tuskegee Syphilis Study from a more humanistic approach rather than from a medical expert's perspective, which has only been the case so far. Interviewing the family members also provides a format in which loved ones can verbally and emotionally express how the syphilis study affected them and their loved ones involved in the study. Such a documentary also provides an effective format for healing and reconciliation. Producers Oprah Winfrey and Alan Ball are scheduled to make an HBO documentary about the book, *The Immortal Life of Henrietta Lacks*, by Rebecca Skloot. The movie will document the life story of Mrs. Lacks as described so vividly in the book. This movie will serve as a beginning point for healing for her family members, who were so tragically affected by the unethical means by which their ancestor's cells were extracted.

5) Lastly, I am in the process of completing a collage series that visually documents the various perspectives, ethical implications, and spiritual manifestations of the Tuskegee Syphilis Study. Some of the art pieces in the series (each 16 by 20 inches) will be included in my master's thesis in bioethics. The collage series will serve as an interpretive model of ethics and

morality in order to visually educate and provoke meaningful discussions for human healing.

In November of 2012, I presented a lecture on teaching about the Tuskegee Syphilis Study through my art collages at the annual meeting of the American Society for Bioethics and Humanities, which was held at the Hyatt Regency Hotel-Capitol Hill, Washington, DC. In addition, many of my art collages were on exhibition during the annual meeting in order to provide a visual understanding of teaching bioethics through art.

Two art collages from the series have been featured in a newsletter and journal in 2013: the Newsletter of the Center for the Study of Science and Religion (the Earth Institute at Columbia University) and the journal, *Academic Medicine*. The publication of these art collages will further educate the general public and bioethics community about many aspects of the Tuskegee Syphilis Study that are not necessarily known. Furthermore, art, in and of itself, creates an environment for healing that no other therapeutic or medical aesthetic can provide.

Concluding Remarks

Philosophy can serve an integral role in resolving historical inequalities, inequities, and injustice in health care. It fosters the discussion of how concepts, theories, and sound reasoning can eventually lead to practical and well-meaning solutions to many of life's deepest ills. In the case of inequality in health care, my paper focused on two philosophical concepts that are not perfect, but nevertheless, serve as building blocks for tangible solutions to health-care disparities in American society. Unethical clinical trials such as the Tuskegee Syphilis Study and the Henrietta Lacks Experiment serve as prevailing examples of how inequities in medicine and health care can promote the occurrence of unethical studies conducted on vulnerable populations.

The systematic encouragement of fairness, justice, and reparations for past misdeeds by the medical establishment aids in decreasing the chances of such injustices occurring again. Tangible initiatives promoting social equality through holistic healing provide real-life solutions to real-life ethical challenges. It is my greatest aspiration to see the fruition of ethical healing initiatives for families affected so dramatically by the unethical experiments involving Mrs. Henrietta Lacks and victims of the Tuskegee Syphilis Study. To me, this paper has served as a starting point for bringing a voice to the voiceless in order to ensure that such atrocities never repeat themselves.

References

US Public Health Service Syphilis Study at Tuskegee, Centers for Disease Control and Prevention (2012). Retrieved from http://www.cdc.gov/tuskegee/faq.htm

Daniels, N. (2012). "Justice, health, and health care," *Medicine and social Justice: Essays on the distribution of health care*, 2nd Edition. Ed. by Rhodes, R., Battin, M., and Silvers, A.) Oxford University Press.

Daniels, N., Kennedy, B. P., and Kawachi, I. (1999). *Why justice is good for our health: The social determinants of health inequalities*. The MIT Press.

Locke, J. (1690). *Two Treatises on Government*. The Project Gutenberg Ebook.

Pollock, J. M. (2005). *The rationale for imprisonment*. The philosophy and history of prisons handbook.

Skloot, R. (2010). *The immortal life of Henrietta Lacks*. The Crown Publishing Group. The National Archives and Records Administration, Southeast Region. (2012). Morrow, Georgia.

Appendices

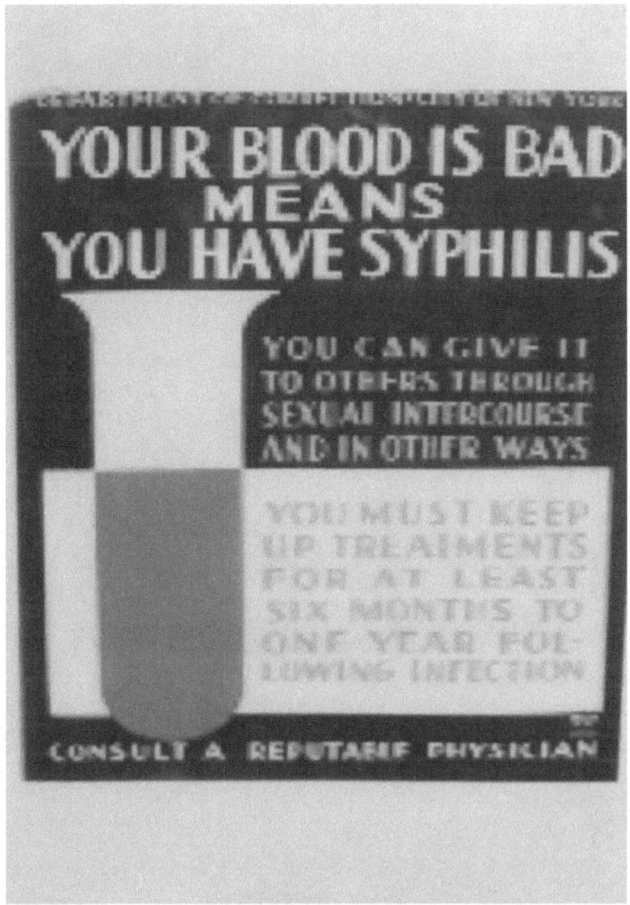

Recruitment and treatment flyer for people who were deemed to have "bad blood," a term used to describe those with syphilis. Source: Photography taken by Obiora N. Anekwe in 2012 at the Legacy Museum, Tuskegee University.

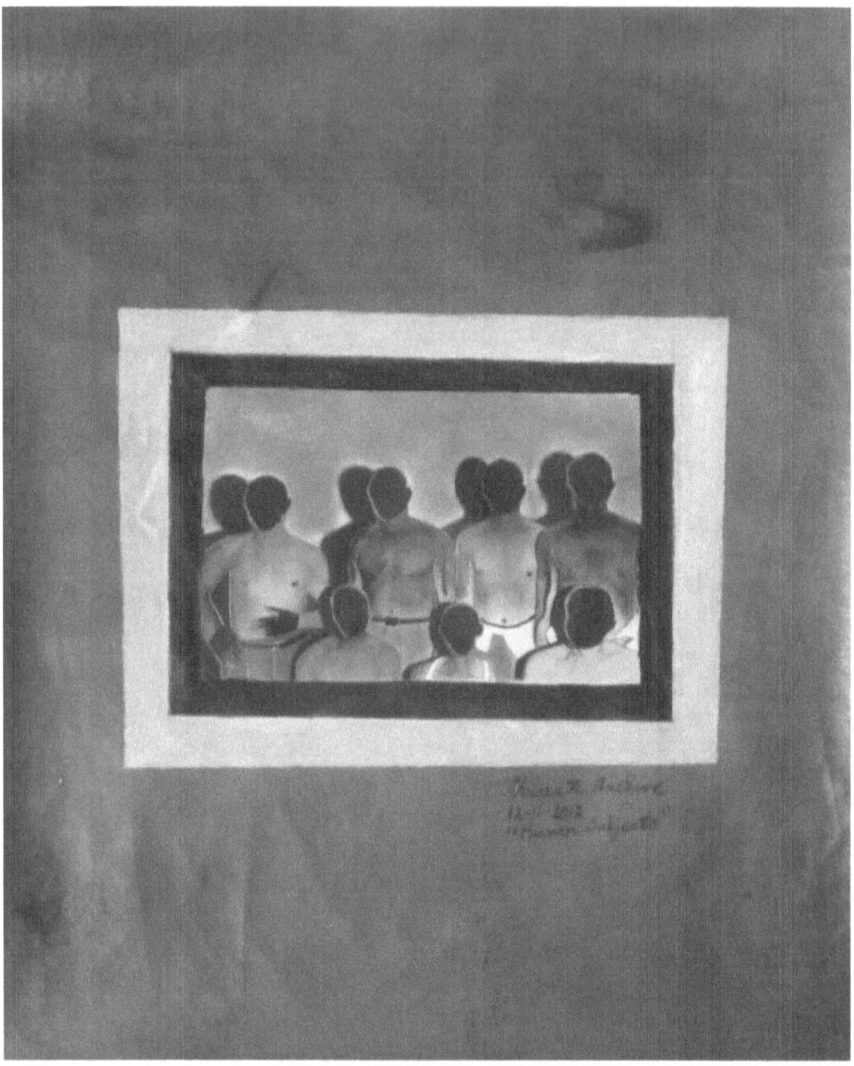

Collage image titled, *Human Subjects*, by Obiora N. Anekwe. The art collage shows seven African-American men who were human subjects in the Tuskegee Syphilis Study. The faces of the men are blackened to represent the concept of being invisible human subjects or guinea pigs experimented upon by public health practitioners. There are black shadows behind each man, representing the wide effect this unethical study had on many black men who do not trust the Public Health Service and, therefore, will not participate in future public health clinical trials. Source: Original black and white courtesy of the National Archives and Records Administration, Southeast Region, Morrow, Georgia.

Charlie W. Pollard, et al v. United States of America, et al (1973)

Obiora N. Anekwe

Introduction

The legal ramifications of *Charlie W. Pollard, et al v. United States of America, et al* (1973) were profound to both law and bioethics. As a legal settlement based on a lawsuit by research participants in the Tuskegee Syphilis Study, it brought forth legal and ethical arguments on informed consent that had not been discussed previously in law and medical ethics. Some scholars even suggest that the medical revelation of the Tuskegee Syphilis Study has been a profound impetus in evolving the field of bioethics. In many ways, the Tuskegee Syphilis Study also acts as a precedent regarding informed consent, even though there is no traditional case law involving the study itself.[1]

My paper will focus on presenting the legal arguments presented in the legal case, the ethical laws and policies influenced by the legal settlement, and, lastly, the lawsuit settlement's compensation plan and additional lawsuit settlement recommendations that I plan to provide within the paper.

Legal Arguments: The Defendants and Plaintiffs

In 1972, after Jean Heller published an article in *The New York Times* about the Tuskegee Syphilis Study, the forty-year clinical trial abruptly ended (See Appendices, Figures 1 and 2). The test subjects later realized that they were involved in an experiment without their full consent and that they had not received treatment for syphilis. A group of survivors, led by Mr. Charlie Pollard (Figure 3), approached Attorney Fred Gray Sr. about a lawsuit against the federal government that financially supported the project and the doctors who performed the medical experiment. Mr. Gray agreed to represent the research study participants in *Charlie W. Pollard, et al v. United States of America, et al,* Civil Action 4126-N (1973). In 1973, the lawsuit quickly ended in a settlement with the study participants. They were collectively awarded ten million dollars that was divided among the living syphilitics/control subjects and families of the deceased. In 1997, President Clinton formally apologized for the Tuskegee Syphilis Study. At the time of the apology, only seven men from the study were living.[2]

On July 24, 1973, the lawsuit was filed with jurisdiction invoked under (1) the Fourth, Fifth, Eighth, Ninth, Thirteenth and Fourteenth Amendments to the US Constitution; (2) the civil rights laws 42 USC Section 1981, Section 1985, Section 2000 (D); (3) the Federal Torts Claims Act, 28 USC 2671; (4) the federal common law; and (5) the Constitution, statutes, and common law of Alabama.[3]

In *Pollard v. United States of America* (1973), Attorney Gray's complaint stated the following:

1) The US government violated the constitutional rights of the participants.

2) The government knew the participants had syphilis and failed to treat them.

3) The Public Health Service failed to fully disclose to the participants that they had syphilis, that they were participating in the study, and that treatment was available for syphilis.

4) The Public Health Service led the participants to believe that they were being properly treated for whatever diseases they had, when, in fact, they were not being meaningfully treated.

5) The Public Health Service failed to obtain the participants' written consents to be a part of the study.

6) The Study was racially motivated and discriminated against African-Americans in that no whites were selected to participate in the Study.

7) There were no rules and regulations governing the Study.[3]

On May 14, 1974, the United States responded to the complaint and stated the following:

1. The action was barred by the statute of limitations.

2. The injuries and damages alleged by the complaint were caused without the fault, carelessness, or negligence on the part of the defendant or any of its agents, servants, or employees acting within the line and scope of their employment.

3. It denied that the injuries and damages to the participants, as alleged in the complaint, were caused by acts of negligence, or carelessness on the part of the government.[3]

The government denied all allegations of the complaint, but admitted that the Tuskegee Syphilis Study began in 1932, that participants were solely African-American, that these participants were in the study, that the study was conducted by the federal government, and that some study participants had died since 1932. The defendants denied that the men's deaths were a result of the Study.[3]

But just as the Nazi doctors involved in unethical experiments during the Holocaust carefully documented their research findings, the doctors who participated in the Tuskegee Syphilis Study also meticulously documented their research through photographs, medical records, correspondence letters, and other transcripts throughout the forty-year clinical trial. Many letters throughout the history of the Tuskegee Syphilis Study document how US Public Health Service officials were aware of the racist elements of the clinical trial, its lack of full disclosure to trial participants, its blatant attempts to mislead trial participants, and the intentional act of withholding treatment for syphilis even when penicillin became available for medical treatment. These documents alone discredit the defendants' legal arguments. Today, the documents chronicling the progression of the Tuskegee Syphilis Study are housed at the National Archives and Records Administration, Southeast Region in Morrow, Georgia, the Tuskegee University Archives in Tuskegee, Alabama, and various other National Archives sites in the Southeast United States.

The fact that these documents exist and were well preserved validates that the Tuskegee Syphilis Study took place. Furthermore, upon detailed analysis of these records, one can also conclude that the health officials involved in the study were quite aware of the unethical implications of their research. In fact, it was well understood by Public Health Service officials and some administrative/medical staff at Tuskegee Institute that initial details regarding the study should be limited to the general public and research study participants in order preserve the continuation of the clinical trial. In other words, if the general public and research participants were initially fully aware of the study's unethical research goals, there would have been a distinct possibility that the study itself would have been criticized and eventually discontinued.

According to Fred Gray Sr., the Tuskegee Syphilis Study was unaffected by the Nuremberg Code and the study continued until the national media exposed the study.[2] Once the study was revealed publicly in 1972, many comparisons to Nazi experiments were made. One US Public Health Service employee wrote a letter to his supervisors describing how "the Tuskegee study could be compared to the German medical 'experiments' at Dachau, and that the Proceedings of the International Military Tribunal in Nuremberg could be used in an attack upon the moral justification for the study."[3] Subsequently, Attorney Gray researched and collected documents from the Nuremberg Trials, along with evidence from the Tuskegee Syphilis Study, which proved that the study was unconstitutional.[2] Using all the information he researched and collected, Attorney Gray proved his allegations, and the case was settled out of court for the Tuskegee Syphilis Study participants.

I believe that an additional legal argument could have been explored by Gray that would have further enhanced his legal argument. My argument centers on the psychological implications of what I describe as *generational suffering*, which emphasizes that the psychological and physical pain that was inflected upon the victims of the clinical trial also systematically affected family members of the victims, such as their wives and children. Syphilis was a disease that not only affected the men involved in the study but was transmitted to the wives of the victims. Furthermore, various psychological impacts of syphilis also affected the victims' children, which could have been clinically documented. These medically known facts about syphilis could have strengthened the plaintiffs' legal arguments, which may have, in the end, greatly enhanced the lawsuit settlement's compensation plan.

Legal Theories of the Settlement

Attorney Gray's legal theory is based on the notion that the tenant farmers selected for the Study were consciously chosen due to their race.[1] As a result of his legal theory, Attorney Gray did not name as defendants the African-American physicians and nurses involved in the study due to the victimization of these professionals by a racially segregated medical profession, which mitigated their legal culpability.[1] Gray believed that race had a greater explanatory factor than aspects of professionalism.[1]

The Tuskegee Syphilis Study implicates two forms of discrimination:

Multiple discrimination can occur in at least two ways: where the grounds of discrimination are additive in nature, and/or where the discrimination is based on an invisible combination of two or more social characteristics. The former, *additive discrimination*, describes a situation where an individual "belongs to two different groups, both of which are affected by [discrimination] practices." The latter, commonly referred to as *intersectional discrimination*, arises out of the combination of various oppressions which, together, produce something unique and distinct from any one form of discrimination standing alone.[4]

In the 1940s, research practices were such that forms of oppression were directed toward black research subjects, promoting race based medical practices. For instance, one New York surgeon in 1926 stated, "The Negro has always been appropriated as choice 'clinical material' by the medical profession. In the eyes of the racists in that profession, the Negro was always next in line beyond the experimental animal."[4] Nonetheless, the African-American men involved in the Tuskegee Syphilis Study were victimized both because of their race and their status as research subjects.[4]

I argue that the legal theory promoted by the plaintiffs' attorney limited full accountability toward the African-American doctors and nurses involved in the study. The exclusion of these medical and health-care officials due to race also hindered the accuracy of the narrative of truth involved in the study. For instance, because the names of the African-American physicians and health-care officials who directly participated in the study were not disclosed but sealed as part of the original lawsuit settlement, many have speculated about the extent of the role the African-American medical staff played in the syphilis study. A greater mystery still lingers regarding the study and a greater mistrust has been engendered toward Tuskegee University medical and administrative staff officials because the Tuskegee Syphilis Study was conducted on the campus of Tuskegee University in the John A. Andrew Memorial Hospital.

Another factor associated with the Tuskegee Syphilis Study is the issue of social and economic class. The African-American doctors who played a role in the study were mostly of the upper-middle-class establishment of Tuskegee, whereas many of the

African-American male study participants were mostly tenant farmers. Although not all the men involved in the study were of a lower social and economic class, a majority of them were. Therefore, the African-American men involved in the study may have been viewed by the African-American physicians and administrative staff as less valuable due to their socioeconomic class. This factor may explain why African-American physicians and medical researchers at Tuskegee University's John A. Andrew Memorial Hospital and other prestigious black universities published reports about the study in medical journals such as the *Journal of the National Medical Association* (JNMA). At the time, the journal served as the forum for research findings by African-American doctors due to the racial segregation practices espoused by the American Medical Association (AMA). An example of a working draft from a research paper on the Tuskegee Syphilis Study can be viewed in the appendices section of this paper (Figure 4).

The final issue associated with the study and lawsuit settlement centers on the issue of education. Most of the African-American men who participated in the study were less formally educated. One participant had a college degree, some men were trained in the industrial arts and farming, and other men owned their own farms. The opportunity to be welcomed onto the campus of Tuskegee University in order to participate in the study was viewed by many people in the community as prestigious and significant. Social and economic issues affected the relationships among African-Americans throughout the City of Tuskegee and Macon County. These factors were not only apparent locally but in the larger African-American community nationwide due to internalized racism and social stratification based on externalized constructs such as complexion.

In Macon County, Alabama, along with most Black Belt counties in the South, health care was not as accessible to many people in the outskirts of the city. The study participants lived mostly in rural areas with less access to health-care facilities such as hospitals and clinics. The John A. Andrew Memorial Hospital represented, to many study participants, the best and nearest facility in Macon County for medical and health-care treatment.

Although the syphilitic men were unaware that they had syphilis, they were aware that they had some kind of medical condition that needed to be treated. These men were misled to believe that they were being treated and cured of "bad blood." Rather they were taken advantage of and used as virtual guinea pigs in an experiment to see how their bodies would react to syphilis until death. When it was learned by the men that free treatment was available to treat their "bad blood," they took the opportunity offered by the US Public Health Service because they thought it represented a step up from the substandard health-care in many Black Belt communities.

Ethical Laws/Policies Established during and after the Tuskegee Syphilis Study

Prior to World War II, no formal protections existed for human subjects in research. In 1948, the Nuremberg Code established ten standards for physicians to conform to when conducting experiments on human participants. These were: 1) volunteers freely consent to participate; 2) researchers fully inform volunteers concerning the study; 3) risks associated with the study are reduced where possible; 4) researchers are responsible for protecting participants against remote harms; 5) participants can withdraw from the study at any time; 6) qualified researchers conduct the study; 7) cessation of the study if adverse effects emerge; 8) society should benefit from study findings; 9) research on humans should be based on previous animal or other previous work; and 10) a research study should never begin if there is a reason to believe that death or injury may result.[5]

The Nuremberg Code developed as a result of judgment by an American military war crimes tribunal conducting proceedings against twenty-three Nazi physicians and administrators for their participation in war crimes and crimes against humanity.[5] These doctors had conducted medical experiments on concentration camp prisoners who later died or were affected as a result. The Nuremberg Code was formed in response to the judicial condemnation of acts of Nazi physicians, but it did not address human subject research in the context of the patient-physician relationship.[5]

It was not until 1964 that the World Medical Association developed ethical principles as guidance for medical doctors in biomedical research involving human subjects, which is known as the Declaration of Helsinki. Until the Declaration of Helsinki, human subject research in the context of the patient-physician relationship had not been addressed.[5] The declaration was formulated in response to concerns about research on patient populations. Its primary purpose was to declare individual patient interests before those of society.[5]

The basic principles of the Declaration of Helsinki are the following: 1) the physician's duty in research is to protect the life, health, privacy, and dignity of the human participant; 2) research involving humans must conform to generally accepted scientific principles and thorough knowledge of scientific literature and methods; 3) research protocols should be reviewed by an independent committee; 4) research protocols should be conducted by medically/scientifically qualified individuals; 5) risks and burden to the participant should not outweigh benefits; 6) researcher should stop study if risks are found to outweigh potential benefits; 7) research is justified only if there is a reasonable likelihood that the population under the study will benefit from the results; 8) participants must be volunteers and informed in the research project; 9) every precaution must be taken to respect privacy, confidentiality, and participant's physical and mental integrity; 10) consent must be obtained from minors, if a child is able to do so; and 11) investigators are obliged to preserve the accuracy of results and negative and positive results should be publicly available.[5]

In 1979, the Belmont Report served as an appropriate response from the bioethical and behavioral sciences research community. Informed consent, assessment of risks and benefits, and selection of research subjects were addressed through the report's three basic ethical principles:

1. Respect for persons, which recognized the autonomy of individuals and the fact that persons with diminished autonomy are entitled to protection.

2. Beneficence, which respects individuals' decisions, protects them from harm, and maximizes possible benefits and minimizes possible harms.

3. Justice, which recognizes that the benefits and risks of research must be distributed fairly.[5]

Due to in large part to the Tuskegee Syphilis Study, these three basic principles have become the foundational principles of modern bioethics in America. Although these principles were not practiced in Tuskegee Syphilis Study, they soon were mandated by the National Research Act of 1974. This act created the Institutional Review Board (IRB), which was formally designated to approve, monitor, and review biomedical and behavioral research involving humans with the aim to protect the rights and welfare of the research subjects.[5]

According to the institutional review board, board members would assist the research investigator in his or her cost-benefit analysis in order to determine whether the use of human subjects was appropriate.[1] Without approval by the IRB, federal funds for the proposed research would be denied. Another aspect of the National Research Act of 1974 was the establishment of the National Commission for the Protection of Human Subjects, which is designed to advise Congress and the executive branch about policies regarding the use of human subjects.[1]

Lawsuit Settlement Compensation Overview

The plaintiffs' complaint, which was filed in the United States District Court for Middle District of Alabama, claimed that the defendants' conduct violated the constitutional rights of the survivors and the deceased participants in the study. Additionally, the complaint requested that each survivor or descendant's representative receive $1.5 million as compensation for the violation of their constitutional rights.[1]

The plaintiffs' lawyers and the United States government reached a monetary settlement in which each surviving victim received $37,500, each heir or representative of the deceased victim was awarded fifteen thousand dollars, each of the control group participants were awarded sixteen thousand dollars, and the heirs or representative of each control group participant received five thousand dollars as a result of the ten-million-dollar settlement paid by the federal government.[1]

Many critics, including family members of victims involved in the syphilis study, have noted that the joint monetary compensation award was insignificant when compared to the physical and mental suffering these victims suffered. It is important to indicate that the money these men and their families received is significantly less than the amount they would have received by today's standard for legal monetary compensation. But more importantly, many victims and their family members never truly benefited from the monetary compensation plan, because the amount of money awarded was so small that it did not pass from generation to generation to benefit future descendants.

Lawsuit Settlement Recommendations

I argue that the settlement reached by the parties involved did not extend far enough to meet the needs of the study participants who died as a result of the nontreatment of syphilis. Therefore, I offer several recommendations that should have been implemented to address the harm suffered by the subjects in the Tuskegee Syphilis Study:

- Accountability by government agencies such as the United States Department of Public Health
- Legal revocation of medical licenses for public health doctors involved in the study
- Human rights violations charges against public health officials involved in the study
- Henceforth, criminal prosecution of public health officials involved in the study based on these human rights violations.

These recommendations are based on current understanding of basic human rights violations that took place during the Tuskegee Syphilis Study. According to Amnesty International in 2011, human rights are basic rights and freedoms that all people are entitled to regardless of nationality, sex, national or ethnic origin, race, religion, language, or any other status.[6] These rights include civil and political rights, such as the right to life, liberty and freedom of expression and social, cultural and economic rights including the right to participate in culture, the right to food, and the right to work and receive an education.[7] Thus, human rights are protected and upheld by international and national laws and treaties. Because the Tuskegee Syphilis Study violated these basic human rights, I assert that all medical and administrative staff involved in the study should be held accountable based the United Nations General Assembly adoption of the Universal Declaration of Human Rights (UDHR) of 1948.

The declaration serves as the foundation of the international system of protection for human rights.[6] The lawsuit settlement did not fully address the human rights violation policies and laws established during the period of the Tuskegee Syphilis Study, which could have held all involved medical parties accountable regardless of race. Rather, the legal theory's foundation was based solely on the medical racism of the white American Public Health Service officials, which ultimately shortchanged the social, educational, and health-care compensation benefits that are necessary to create holistic healing from the wrongs suffered during the study.

The monetary compensation provided to the syphilis study participants was too limited and distracted from the primary purpose of health care and medicine, which is healing. Monetary compensation was the primary vehicle for providing healing to the study participants and family members. But other means of compensation should have be considered, such as the development of health-care facilities and hospitals in the Macon County community and the establishment of educational development initiatives for the study participants and their family members that would help eliminate health-care disparities in Black Belt communities. Nevertheless, the larger issues of mental and physical healing have yet to be fully acknowledged, confronted and settled as a result of the alleged anguish, pain, and suffering many of these men faced as a result of their participation in the study.

Nonetheless, I contend that providing governmental compensation to victims is just one response to the persistent public-health and bioethical challenge of human experimentation. In future legal bioethical cases, other responses must be considered in the progressive movement toward a conceptualization of the social functions of science, medicine, and law.

Concluding Remarks

The legal and ethical responses to the Tuskegee Syphilis Study demonstrate the lack of humane and ethical experimentation practices that occurred among vulnerable populations based on race, class, and health-care disparities before the 1970s. As a consequence, the dominant lesson that emerges from the lawsuit settlement and its efforts to eliminate race-based medical practice centers on a continued effort to emphasize the constitutive nature of human equality.

Although the lawsuit settlement did not provide the results that may have led to greater healing for study participants and accountability for the health-care staff involved in the Tuskegee Syphilis Study, its results provided a benchmark for informed consent policies that did not exist prior to the lawsuit settlement. As future bioethicists, it is our duty to shed light on the unethical medical and health-care practices of the past in order to correct them for future generations to ensure that these unethical practices do not occur again.

Endnotes

[1] Palmer, L. I. (1997). "Paying for suffering: The problem of human experimentation," *Faculty Publications*. Paper 533. Retrieved from http://scholarship.law.wm.edu/facpubs

[2] www.history.ucsb.edu. *The Tuskegee syphilis study.*

[3] Gray, F. D. (1998). *The Tuskegee syphilis study.* Montgomery, Alabama: New South Books.

[4] Hunter, N. D. (2010). "Rights talk and patient subjectivity: The role of autonomy, equality, and participation norms," *Wake Forest Law Review*, Vol. 45.

[5] University of Waterloo. (2011). "Research with humans." Retrieved from www.iris.waterloo.ca/ethics/human/resource/index.htm

[6] "African-American Trailblazers in Virginia History" (2011). Retrieved from http://www.lva.virginia.gov/public/trailblazers/2011/lacks.htm

[7] Amnesty International USA. (2011). "Basic human rights." Retrieved from www.amnestyusa.org/research/human-rights-basics

Appendices

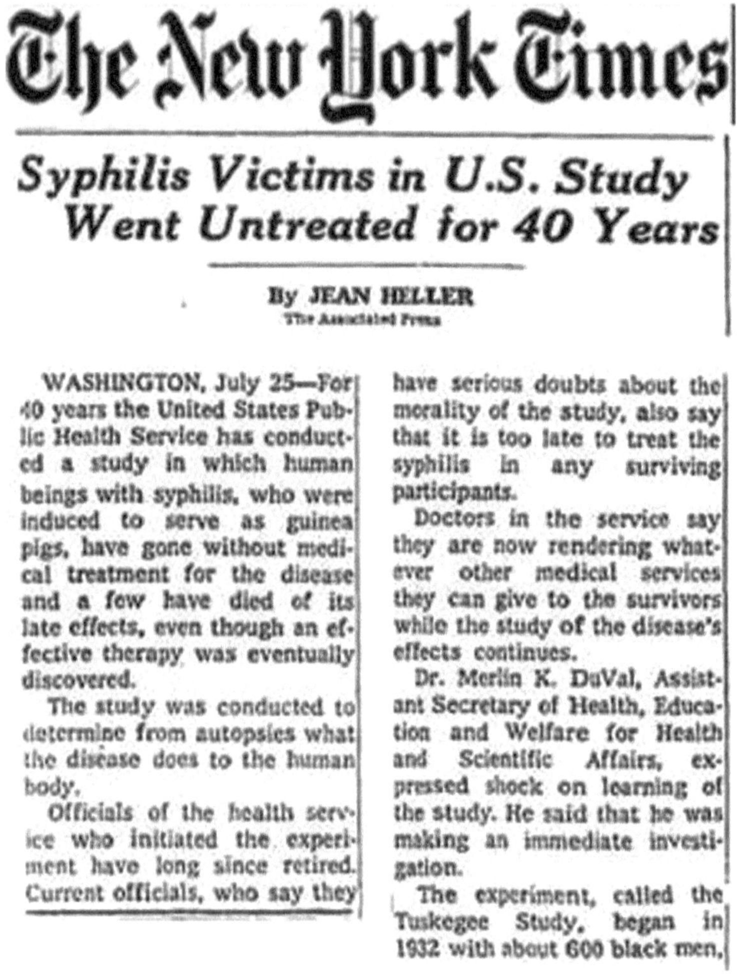

The New York Times

Syphilis Victims in U.S. Study Went Untreated for 40 Years

By JEAN HELLER
The Associated Press

WASHINGTON, July 25—For 40 years the United States Public Health Service has conducted a study in which human beings with syphilis, who were induced to serve as guinea pigs, have gone without medical treatment for the disease and a few have died of its late effects, even though an effective therapy was eventually discovered.

The study was conducted to determine from autopsies what the disease does to the human body.

Officials of the health service who initiated the experiment have long since retired. Current officials, who say they have serious doubts about the morality of the study, also say that it is too late to treat the syphilis in any surviving participants.

Doctors in the service say they are now rendering whatever other medical services they can give to the survivors while the study of the disease's effects continues.

Dr. Merlin K. DuVal, Assistant Secretary of Health, Education and Welfare for Health and Scientific Affairs, expressed shock on learning of the study. He said that he was making an immediate investigation.

The experiment, called the Tuskegee Study, began in 1932 with about 600 black men.

Figure 1: The article by Jean Heller that uncovered the forty-year syphilis study. Source: Heller, J. (1972), *The New York Times*.

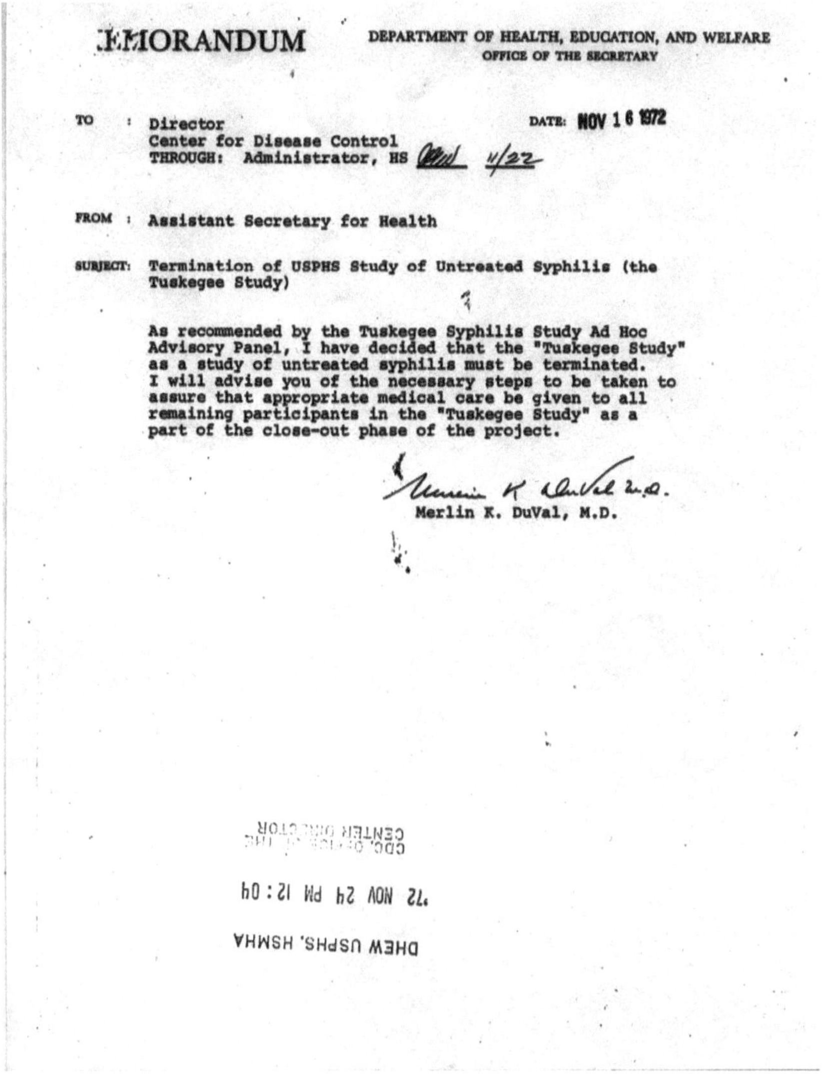

.EMORANDUM   DEPARTMENT OF HEALTH, EDUCATION, AND WELFARE
OFFICE OF THE SECRETARY

TO   : Director   DATE: NOV 16 1972
          Center for Disease Control
          THROUGH: Administrator, HS

FROM : Assistant Secretary for Health

SUBJECT: Termination of USPHS Study of Untreated Syphilis (the
          Tuskegee Study)

          As recommended by the Tuskegee Syphilis Study Ad Hoc
          Advisory Panel, I have decided that the "Tuskegee Study"
          as a study of untreated syphilis must be terminated.
          I will advise you of the necessary steps to be taken to
          assure that appropriate medical care be given to all
          remaining participants in the "Tuskegee Study" as a
          part of the close-out phase of the project.

                                    Merlin K. DuVal, M.D.

                    CENTER DIRECTOR
                    CDC OFFICE OF THE

                    '72 NOV 24 PM 12:04

                    DHEW USPHS, HSMHA

Figure 2: The memorandum that formally abruptly ended the Tuskegee Syphilis Study.
Source: The National Archives and Records Administration, Southeast Region, Morrow,
Georgia.

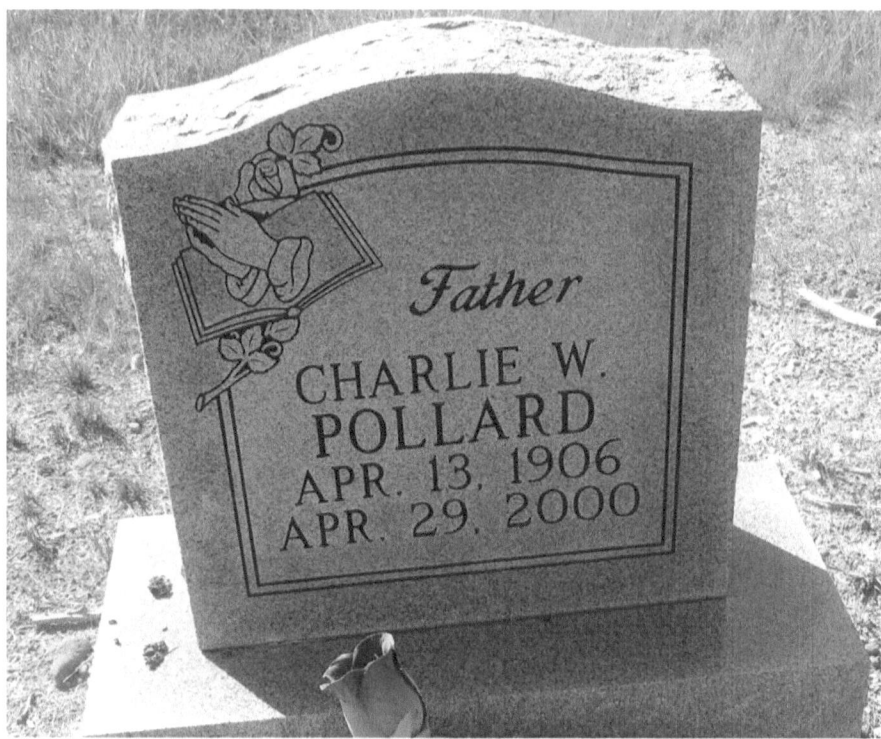

Figure 3: Photograph of Charles W. Pollard's burial headstone, the lead plaintiff in the legal settlement for victims of the Tuskegee Syphilis Study. Location: Shiloh Cemetery site in Notasulga, Alabama. Photographer: Obiora N. Anekwe

Figure 4: A sample research paper on the Tuskegee Syphilis Study. Source: The National Archives and Records Administration, Southeast Region, Morrow, Georgia.

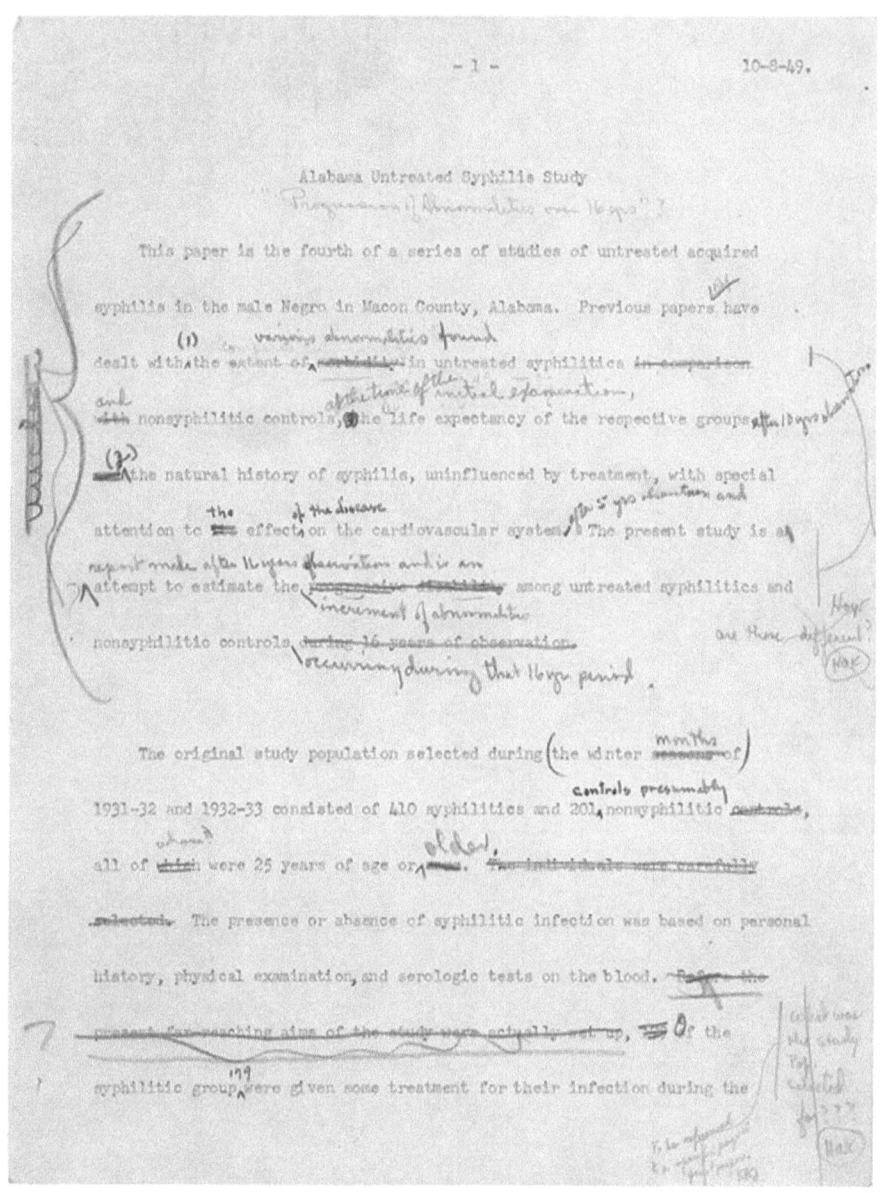

- 2 -

period of this first examination. Most of these individuals were among the

younger age groups, and were given amounts of treatment varying from 1 to 15

shots of neoarsephenamine. *These have been dropped from consideration in the present paper* A second complete physical examination was made

of the majority of the group in 1938-39. ~~However, no strenuous effort was made~~

~~to locate those who had received treatment, and consequently a large number of~~

~~them lapsed from observation.~~ Since 1939, there has been an annual visit to

Macon County by a physician for the purpose of obtaining specimens of blood for

serologic examination. In the fall of 1948 a third physical examination was

performed on the individuals who could be located at that time, ~~again with no~~

~~particular emphasis on those who had received some treatment.~~

An important phase of the study has been the performance of autopsies on

the individuals who have died. Through 1948, ~~162~~ *140* of the number included in the

original population have died, and of these ~~113~~ *98* have been autopsied. Of those *m*

autopsies have not been performed,
who ~~have not been autopsied,~~ proof of death has been established by death

certificate or by information furnished by relatives or friends of the deceased.

Because of the relatively non-migratory nature of the group, it is reasonably

certain that there have been no other deaths than the ~~162~~ *140* recorded. No analysis

of autopsy data will be attempted in this report; a detailed account of this

Truth Telling: Ancestral Voices Rising Up from the USPHS Syphilis Study in Tuskegee

Obiora N. Anekwe
and
Ejinkonye C. Anekwe

Authors' Note

The opinions expressed in this article are those of the authors alone, and not of the educational institutions they represent. The authors express solemn thanks to the family members of the men who were enrolled in the USPHS Syphilis Study in Tuskegee. The article is dedicated to their struggles with unethical human experimentation and the attempt at reconciliation through former President Clinton's 1997 apology. In addition, the authors thank their mother, Emma Jeanette Anekwe, for encouraging them to conduct research on the syphilis study. The authors were born in the 1970s at the John A. Andrew Memorial Hospital, where the syphilis study was conducted in part. They also hold masters degrees from Tuskegee University, class of 1999. Both authors were in attendance at Tuskegee University in 1997, the year President Clinton issued his apology to the survivors of the study. The first author took all photographs. Despite the apology, the consequences of the experiment at Tuskegee are far-reaching in the United States. The study is significant to the authors, because they were both born in the hospital where the experiment was conducted. The authors wish to develop an initiative of holistic healing both to confront the past and understand how to assuage the descendants' pain. As holistic healing acts as a comforter for them, its greater goal is to honor the sacrifices of their ancestors and to offer ways to gain hope for the future.

Abstract

Medical researcher and virologist Jonas Salk once stated, "Our greatest responsibility is to be good ancestors." His words reflect the belief that we are ethically responsible and universally connected to our communal family. Reactions to medical experiments such as the US Public Health Service Syphilis Study in Tuskegee can serve as examples in how truth telling can reinforce ethical measures to protect human subjects in clinical research and how to interpret the ancestral voices of former syphilis experiment participants to promote positive change and create an environment of holistic healing for families damaged by such studies. The analysis concentrates on the concepts of doctor-patient relationship, truth telling, informed consent, patient rights, end-of-life care, and ethical implications of clinical coercion and deception. What emerges is a model of effective truth telling that informs the doctor-patient relationship, creates a greater awareness of ethical medical practices, and promotes an environment of healing over harm.

Keywords: truth telling, informed consent, holistic healing, participant, family, syphilis study, Tuskegee

Introduction

The United States Public Health Service Syphilis Study was conducted in Tuskegee, Alabama, from 1932 to 1972 (Shakir, 2011a). Also known at times as the Tuskegee Study of Untreated Syphilis in the Negro Male, the intent of the research was to ascertain the extent to which syphilis, in its untreated state, affected the physiology of African-American males. Participants in the study included 399 African-American men with late stage syphilis and 201 African-American men who were uninfected with syphilis. The latter served as a control group for the symptomatic participants (Centers for Disease Control and Prevention, 2011).

The ethical grounding of the experiment was ill-conceived and violated the human rights of the patients on many levels. Scientists did not tell the patients the nature of their illness but that they had "bad blood," which was a colloquial term for a variety of unrelated ailments (Shakir, 2011a). It was an act of deceit. As the experiment progressed, the venereal disease took its natural course and the men were unaware of the danger (Shakir, 2011a). The scientists took great pains to restrict the men from seeking any form of treatment, including penicillin, which was proven to treat syphilis successfully (Shakir, 2011a). See Photograph 1 below for a depiction of related but unused treatment drugs. The study continued to take place in Tuskegee until 1972. President Clinton offered an official apology in 1997 (Shakir, 2011a), but the healing and education must continue.

Operational Definitions: Family and Informed Consent

Family is defined as a unit consisting of at least one parent, at least one offspring, and which may include relatives such as aunts, uncles, and grandparents. The parameters of this definition are loose because many African-Americans are raised in extended, multigenerational families, unlike the stereotypical nuclear family, which consists of a mother, a father, and siblings. Throughout the African-American experience, including today, it is not uncommon for children to be raised in a single-parent family with grandparents and other relatives due to kinship and/or socioeconomic reasons.

Informed consent usually refers to consent that a person gives that meets certain minimum standards. Further, an informed consent can be given based upon a clear understanding of the facts, implications, and future consequences of an action. To provide truly *informed* consent, the person involved in a study must have adequate reasoning faculties and be in possession of relevant facts at the time consent is given (Berg, Appelbaum,

Parker, and Lidz, 2001). Impairments in reasoning and judgment such as basic intellectual/emotional immaturity, high levels of stress, severe mental illness, intoxication, severe sleep deprivation, Alzheimer's disease, or being in a coma constitute examples of impaired consent. The term *informed consent* was first used in the 1957 medical malpractice case by attorney Paul G. Gebhard (Solomon, 2006).

Truth telling is very important to this study. It is a communication of facts in a manner in which a patient should be able to understand them (Kirklin, 2007, p. 11). Telling the truth to people who may not understand certain conditions is challenging. Often there is a conundrum over telling the truth and protecting patients from harm (Kirklin, 2007, p. 11). For example, Kirklin (2007) stated that the use of honesty is controversial because of competing moral necessities, such as avoiding harm. However, many researchers suggest that doctors should tell the truth (Kirklin, 2007, p. 11). Truth telling may even involve the use of metaphor as a means of communication to patients who lack the professional or personal experience to make a comparison to the conditions that they have (Kirklin, 2007, p. 11).

Definition and Applications of Illness and Healing

Illness

A brief definition of illness should precede a definition of holistic healing. Illness has been described as an experience that affects the body and soul (Meyerstein, 2005). Diseases bring about a number of symptoms that can be described as illnesses (Meyerstein, 2005). When people experience illness, they undergo physical changes, as well as fear of losing control (Meyerstein, 2005). Illness can take people into unknown territory, often leading to feelings of isolation. The patient is bombarded by issues of medical treatment while receiving limited attention to the spiritual and emotional aspects of dealing with illnesses (Meyerstein, 2005).

Illness does not encompass only physical symptoms, but mental symptoms as well. Depression, for instance, may be characterized as an illness by Western medical standards. According to Storck, Csordas, and Milton (2000), depression is classified as an illness in the American Psychiatric Association's 1994 Diagnostic and Statistical Manual of Mental Disorders, Fourth Edition (DSM-IV) and the The International Classification of Diseases-Tenth Edition (ICD-10) (World Health Organization 1991) (Storck, Csordas, and Milton, 2000, p. 573). In order for someone to be diagnosed with depression according to both ICD and DSM-IV standards, one must exhibit low mood and/or a disinterest in hobbies and activities for a minimum of two weeks. In addition, a person with depression may experience appetite changes, sleep pattern changes, reduced concentration, and bouts of fatigue (Storck, Csordas, and Milton, 2000, p. 573).

The use of the DSM-IV and ICD as diagnostic tools for psychiatric illnesses are seen as restrictive and offer no treatment strategy (Storck et al, 2000, p. 573). Tucker (1998), as quoted in Storck et al (2000), believed that the DSM-IV and ICD ignore the history of the patient, and instead, focuses on just diagnosis, which Tucker saw as reductionist (Storck et al, 2000, p. 573). However, Storck et al (2000), citing Engels (1980), believed that if healers are to be successful, their diagnosis of illness must include psychological, somatic, and cultural factors (Storck et al, 2000, p. 573).

Healing

Healing, in general, involves access to remedies that can place a patient on the path to wellness. Modern notions of healing date back to the thirteenth century, when the physician Zohar suggested that physicians should give medicine to help their patients. For instance, wishing someone *refuah sheleymah* means to wish someone a full recovery of body and spirit (Meyerstein, 2005). Thus, even before the advent of modern medicine, some people believed that healing involved both physical and spiritual cleansing.

Healing does not necessarily always mean a physical cure to a physical ailment. Healing can involve sharing individual or group life stories. Oral history is used in Africa to convey actions, such as those of royal persons (Schoenbrun, 2006). These oral histories allow members of diverse communities to establish friendships. In Uganda there is an oral tradition about a large group of women who offer coffee berries and cash to a grandmother-like spirit guide known as a *jjaajja* so that they might be blessed with a better job or other forms of good fortune (Scboenbrun, 2006). This spiritual ritual took place at a shrine located on a hill on the outskirts of Kampala. The jjajja dances through fire, unharmed. After the ceremony is over, the followers then travel to the shores of Lake Victoria in order to meet the jjajja at her house where she tattoos them. Later they proceed to confess their transgressions. Finally, the jjajja gives them coffee berries to swallow (Scboenbrun, 2006).

The significance of this particular oral tradition is interesting. The spiritual journey of the participants is symbolic of colonial practices of capitalism, kinship, and royalty (Scboenbrun, 2006). The oral tradition of the jjajja emphasizes the hybridization of African and Western cultures. The notion of the unburned jjajja is not unique to Uganda. It is found throughout the African Great Lakes. Schoenbrun (2006) mentioned that people in Rwanda believe in the same spirit. Also, coffee beans are exchanged as a form of kinship in the Great Lakes Region (Scboenbrun, 2006).

In addition to oral traditions, prayer healing is used in both traditional and modern societies to cure ailments. For example, traditional healers are an accepted part of Iranian society. According to Javaheri (2006), prayer is common in all religious systems (Javaheri, 2006, p. 172). Javaheri (2006), citing Eliade (1987), stated that prayer, as a human communication with divine entities, has been present in most religions throughout history (Javaheri, 2006, p. 172). Javaheri (2006), citing Grant (1995), also stated that prayer has been known to function in invocation, adoration, confession of sin, and thanksgiving (Javaheri, 2006, p. 172). In addition, prayer may manifest itself as active or passive prayer, private versus corporate, formal versus free prayer, or direct versus indirect prayer (Javaheri, 2006, p. 172).

Prayer used by a form of healing in a special way is referred to as prayer healing. According to Easthope (1998), as cited by Javaheri (2006), prayer healing can be classified as a form of alternative medicine. Prayer healing, or spiritual healing, includes faith healing, counseling, energy therapy, and transcendental meditation (Javaheri, 2006, p. 172). Javaheri (2006) takes great care to distinguish between spirituality and religion. Religion, stated Javaheri, is based on doctrines and belief systems regarding the essence of God and how He relates to humanity. Spirituality, on the other hand, is concerned about common experiences underlying religious concepts and how it relates to humanity (Javaheri, 2006, p. 172).

Prayer healing in Iran has its roots in ancient faiths such as the Zoroastrian religion, as well as Islam (Javaheri, 2006, p. 172). For instance, several verses in the Qur'an, the Holy Scriptures of Muslims, dictate the importance of spiritual healing. One such verse, Verse 82 of Chapter Bani-Israel, refers to the Qur'an as a means of healing (Javaheri, 2006, p. 172). Prayer in Muslim cultures is very formal and all Muslims must pray five times a day. Despite this formality, informal ways of prayer exist. For instance, prayer can be used to solve problems. In Shiite Muslim culture, followers pray to the Prophet as well as revered imams. One site, the shrine of the Eighth Imam in the Iranian city of Mashhad, is a place where practitioners bring their sick loved ones and pray for healing. Such prayer lasts for several days or weeks (Javaheri, 2006, p. 173).

Another aspect of spiritual healing is the role of secular institutions in providing such services. Whereas some places offer spiritual healing through religious institutions, insurance companies in the Netherlands pay for pilgrimages to the Marian Shrine of Lourdes. According to Houtman and Macini (2002), as cited in Notermans (2007), 60 percent of Dutch society identified themselves as secular in 2002, compared to 24 percent in 1958. Many churches in the Netherlands stand empty, while the Dutch government decides whether to redevelop the properties as commercial ventures or landmarks. However, the number of Dutch pilgrimages to Lourdes remains high. In 2007, eleven thousand pilgrims traveled to Lourdes from the Netherlands (Notermans, 2007, p. 217).

A total of six insurance companies pay for pilgrimages to the Marian holy site, with eighteen hundred annual pilgrims using the services of these companies. Some public officials decry the use of insurance money for these pilgrimages, because they believe the trips are not scientifically proven to cure disease. Also, these critics say that the pilgrimages play on people's irrational aspirations for miracles (Notermans, 2007, p. 218). Despite these criticisms, proponents of pilgrimages feel that these ventures are not meant to be understood at the biomedical level; rather, they address loss and pain. Whereas in the past, churches offered hope, the lack of churches necessitate the use of ventures to Lourdes as a way of dealing with the occurrence of pain (Notermans, 2007, p. 218).

Another aspect to spiritual healing is the number of people who reported being healed. According to Poloma and Hoelter (1998), citing studies by Bromley et al (1986), Trier and Shupe (1991), and Poloma and Pendleton (1991), found that 10 percent of respondents experienced healing through prayer (Poloma and Hoelter,

1998, p. 257). Also, in a 1996 Gallup poll, 33 percent of born-again Christians reported being physically healed, compared to only 14 percent of non-born-agains. In addition, 32 percent of born-again Christians were healed from emotional illness, compared to 15 percent of non-born-agains (Poloma and Hoelter, 1998, p. 263). Furthermore, authors such as Deepak Chopra, Larry Dorsey, and Herbert Benson promote the use of spiritual healing as a major component of health (Poloma and Hoelter, 1998, p. 257). Thus, previous research indicates a possible link between spirituality and physical healing (Poloma and Hoelter, 1998, p. 257).

Definition and Application of the Holistic Person and Healing
Holistic healing can be understood in terms of understanding the concept of the holistic person. Riches (2000) referred to understanding the holistic person as one in which the mind is as important as the body (Riches, 2000). The holistic person, as analyzed by Riches, is different from the person who adheres to Western medicine, who was described as a duality consisting of passive body with a soul added to it (Riches, 2000). The movement toward the holistic person has been particularly prominent among feminists and new age practitioners. Feminists believe that Western education has essentially made menopause clinical and mechanized, thereby ignoring the complexity of menopause as an event of change. Feminists, therefore, believe that menopause should be approached from a holistic perspective (Riches, 2000).

New age practitioners regard the person as a combination of physical, spiritual, emotional, and mental attributes (Riches, 2000). The state of well-being is considered equilibrium between the mind and the body. As such, new age believers have an assumption that the human body is capable of self-healing (Riches, 2000). Thus, healing may involve providing remedies to both the body and the spirit of the human being.

Holistic healing may involve several aspects. One such aspect is holistic health care. Marciano (2001) described holistic health care as a field that looks at the mind and spirit as inseparable from the body. As such, all of these factors should be considered as part of the patient's overall care (Marciano, 2001, p. 24A). Marciano also stated that holistic health care is becoming integrated into Western medicine (Marciano, 2001, p. 24A). Governing holistic health care is holistic ethics. Holistic ethics, as cited in Marciano (2001) by Keagan (1995), is described as a set of principles by which one lives their lives. By acting in an ethical manner, one is acting not according to law or social standards, but to help in the process of unity. The person who is striving for unity is doing so based on their character and their relationship to the universe (Marciano, 2001, p. 24A). Mariano (2001), citing Keagan (1995), stated that holistic ethics are based on several tenets:

1. A divine spirit is involved with humanity and the universe.

2. The material world plays only a small part in the divine plan.

3. People have a dual nature, one that is material, and one that is divine.

4. Humanity's purpose is to evolve itself and the universe into a perfect whole.

5. Unity is the fundamental concept in lighting the path of critical wisdom.

6. There is a divine plan for the universe, although it is beyond comprehension. Everything and every action, good or bad, simple or complex, wanted or unwanted, is integral to the divine plan.

7. Adversity can be our greatest teacher.

8. Because each person is part of the greater whole, each moral action affects not just the individual, but humankind.

9. Ethical actions are judged by how they foster wholeness. (Marciano, 2001, 24B-24C)

Thus, holistic ethics encompasses the good that humans can do to each other to foster greater physical and spiritual health.

The USPHS Syphilis Study's Legacy:
Distrust and Harm

The USPHS Syphilis Study at Tuskegee began as a quest to understand the natural progression of the venereal disease. In 1908, the US Congress opened the PHS's Division of Venereal Diseases (Cook and Jackson, 2012). Doctors from the USPHS believed in the prevailing theory that African-Americans manifested symptoms of syphilis differently from Caucasians. To prove that theory, the doctors wished to use a sample of infected black males in Macon County, Alabama, study the natural course of syphilis in this select group, and deny medical treatment (Cook and Jackson, 2012). To exacerbate matters, the men were not told that they were part of a scientific study (Cook and Jackson, 2012).

The event is significant because, as found by Shakir (2011a), the study is still shrouded in silence. Tied to that silence is a great deal of secrecy, and secrecy promotes distrust (Shakir, 2011a). Further, Shakir (2011a) found that women in Macon County and Tuskegee felt embarrassed and ashamed about what happened (Shakir, 2011a). Also troubling is the number of people who know that the experiment existed. When sampling a group of local women, Shakir (2011a) discovered that 67 percent of the group was not familiar with the study (Shakir, 2011a). These findings are particularly disturbing since most women in the group were adults when the experiment was uncovered (Shakir, 2011a).

The study had an impact on the use of the word *Tuskegee*. The name is associated with an internationally famous university, but the word *Tuskegee* is often a metonym for unethical human experimentation in general. Shavers, Lynch, and Burmeister

(2000) strengthen this notion as they explain how the experiment might have contributed to the reluctance of many African-Americans to participate in medical research. Besides the familiar understanding of the mechanics of the experiment, the authors mentioned that the experiment created a backlash from the African-American community (Shavers, Lynch, and Burmeister, 2000, p. 564). Though medical research has not illustrated any correlation between African-American reluctance regarding medical research and the study at Tuskegee (Shavers et al, 2000, p. 564) it does not change the emotional impact of this atrocity on society. Based on this assessment, various researchers sought to find a link between ethnic differences in knowledge of the incident at Tuskegee and the willingness to participate in medical research (Shavers et al, 2000, p. 564).

These researchers interviewed 179 African-American and Caucasian-American residents of Metropolitan Detroit as part of a survey administered through the telephone and the mail (Shavers et al, 2000, p. 563). Statistical analysis was performed using Survey Data Analysis Program Version 7.5 (SUDAAN). Chi-square analysis was used to analyze any differences between groups. In addition, the study was two-tailed, and a significance of 0.05 was used (Shavers et al, 2000, p. 566).

The results indicated that 46 percent of the respondents were African-American, while 46 percent were Caucasian-American. In addition, 81 percent of African-Americans have heard of the USPHS Syphilis Study, compared to 21 percent of Caucasian-Americans (Shavers et al, 2000, p. 566). Furthermore, more African-Americans (54 percent) than Caucasian-Americans (17 percent) had less trust in medical researchers because of their prior knowledge of the USPHS experiment at Tuskegee (Shavers et al, 2000, p. 567). The study confirmed what the researchers already believed: more African-Americans were distrustful of participating in medical research than Caucasians.

Other researchers, such as Fairchild and Bayer (1999), mentioned that the syphilis experiment at Tuskegee is a reason why African-Americans distrust the medical establishment. *Tuskegee* is also a symbol for the greater legacy of slavery, discrimination, and injustice that African-Americans have long endured (Fairchild and Bayer, 1999). The legacy is often compounded by both fact and fiction. For instance, were the unwilling participants of the study given syphilis? Were they denied penicillin as a treatment for syphilis? What happened to the bodies of the participants prior to burial? To answer these questions involves complicated detective work.

Men Were Not Intentionally Infected

Contrary to popular belief, the men were not forcefully given syphilis. According to Reverby (2001), the high levels of syphilis in the area attracted the attention of the USPHS (Reverby, 2001). The rumors of forced injections persisted through the years and are found in talk shows, news broadcasts, and even an Eddie Murphy comedy routine (Reverby, 2001). Reverby noted that the injection myth was expanded to include the Tuskegee Airmen, because the World War II project that they participated in was also called the Tuskegee Experiment. Reverby stated that some people confused the two events, which occurred at the same point in time. It is also interesting that two separate HBO movies about the Tuskegee Airmen and the syphilis study starred the same actor, Lawrence Fishburne. That association may have sparked some confusion on the part of viewers regarding the USPHS study at Tuskegee (Reverby, 2001).

Men Were Denied Treatment

As for the denial of treatment to the study participants, it is certainly true that the men were ill informed about the purpose of the study. They were told they were being treated for "bad blood," and they were denied treatment for syphilis in an organized, intentional effort, even after penicillin was shown to effectively treat syphilis (Fairchild and Bayer, 1999). The USPHS blacklisted the men, adding them to lists that blocked them from seeking treatment from clinics throughout the United States (Shakir, 2011a). USPHS doctors deliberately withheld penicillin from the men based on the argument that administering the antibiotic would be ineffective in the treatment of late-stage syphilis. Unfortunately, the doctors at the USPHS felt that denial of treatment to the men would not cause a moral crisis if penicillin or another treatment were improved (Shakir, 2011a). It is important to note that even though denial of treatment was the norm for the USPHS doctors involved, some men sought and received treatment outside of official USPHS channels.

For example, Reverby (2001) explained that one Tuskegee doctor, Dr. Robert Story, used penicillin to treat men with what he described as "nonsyphilitic" illnesses. He ended up "accidentally" treating patients from the syphilis study (Reverby, 2001, p. 24). In addition to Dr. Story, two doctors who participated in the USPHS Syphilis Study, Dr. Eugene Dibble of John Andrew Memorial Hospital, and Dr. Murray Smith of the Macon County Health Department, "accidentally" treated study participants by giving them penicillin for back pain and other symptoms unrelated to syphilis (Reverby, 2001). Patient records indicate that approximately one-third of the men who secretly received penicillin were administered the drug by either Dr. Dibble or Dr. Smith (Reverby, 2001).

Study participants who did not receive treatment in Tuskegee were referred by Drs. Dibble and Smith to Birmingham's syphilis rapid clinics, although during the early stages of syphilis treatment in the 1940s and 1950s, men with late-stage syphilis were denied treatment (Reverby, 2001). Some participants moved to other parts of the country as part of the great migration out of the American South. In their new homes, the participants struggled to get health care while federal authorities were trying to catch up with them. Despite their best efforts, the USPHS could not prevent all of them from receiving penicillin. In fact, medical records from the 1970s reveal that of the 71 study participants (21 percent) moved from Alabama during the study. Many of these men sought and received treatment for syphilis outside the State of Alabama (Reverby, 2001).

The experiment continued even after the participants died. Their bodies were studied to ascertain the extent of damage done by late-stage syphilis (Cook and Jackson, 2012). Still, questions persist concerning the fate of the remains of the study participants prior to burial. According to Reverby (2001), autopsies were indeed performed on the men at John Andrew Memorial Hospital in Tuskegee (Reverby, 2001). There are cases, however, where some families refused to allow autopsies to be performed on their male relatives (Reverby, 2001).

Brief History of Human Experimentation in the United States of America

Was the USPHS Syphilis Study the only study that used socially marginalized populations in the United States? No. The history of human experimentation in this country can be traced to the 1840s, during slavery. One of the first human experiments involved the use of female African-American slaves for gynecologic surgical procedures. According to Lederer (2005), Dr. James Marion Sims, an Alabama doctor, was approached by local slave-owners who were concerned that their female slaves were suffering from physical complications due to childbirth. Such complications included chronic pain, irritation, and offensive odors emanating from either a ruptured rectum or a bladder (Lederer, 2005, p. 20). Initially disgusted by the thought of treating gynecologic diseases, Dr. Sims became interested as he saw multiple cases of slave mothers with these conditions. Dr. Sims wanted the women's conditions to improve so that they could become more productive. Thus, he convinced owners to allow their female slaves to become patients. In turn, Dr. Sims provided the women with room and board (Lederer, 2005, p. 20).

Dr. Sims operated on the women without anesthesia. He performed at least thirty surgeries on the patients. He admired their ability to remain stoic despite the pain. His research eventually led to effective surgical treatments for gynecologic problems, thus earning his place as one of the pioneers of gynecology in the United States. Dr. Sims was also known as a doctor to both slaves and free people (Lederer, 2005, p. 20). However, many people did not question the use of slaves as test subjects.

Several decades later, another group of socially marginalized people, orphans, were subjected to human experimentation. By the early twentieth century, many doctors and researchers were beginning to understand the importance of employing ethical guidelines to human subject testing. When researching a cure for Yellow Fever in Cuba, Dr. Walter Reed devised written contracts between human subjects and doctors to ensure that the former were not exploited by the latter (Lederer, 2005, p. 21). Also, Progressive-era proponents attempted to enact ethical guidelines to protect patients from unethical experiments. However, many of their recommendations were ignored by state and federal authorities. For example, doctors argued that ethical guidelines would restrict their efforts to make medical progress. Also, the doctors believed that the research did not result in harm to the patients (Lederer, 2005, p. 21).

One questionable research study was conducted in 1910 at the Hebrew Orphan Asylum in New York City. At this facility, orphans were used as patients in an effort to study the effects of scurvy and rickets. In the study, children were denied orange juice in order to ascertain if they developed scurvy. The children exhibited swollen gums, which is one of the symptoms of scurvy. The children were then administered orange juice to see if the symptoms of the disease were reversed (Lederer, 2005, p. 21). The study was heavily criticized by the American press. In response, the physicians stated that the children were not harmed. Also, the doctors felt that the orphans' participation in the study was part of their repayment to society for their care (Lederer, 2005, p. 21). In addition to orphans, prisoners, mental patients, and immigrants were often used as test subjects.

The USPHS Syphilis Study was perhaps the most famous study that involved American test subjects. Originally the study was to last from six months to a year. However, the researchers felt that the most pertinent information concerning the symptoms of syphilis could only be gathered through a thorough, postmortem examination of the test subjects. As a result, the study continued from 1932 to 1972, a period of forty years (Lederer, 2005, p. 21). By the end of the 1960s, scientists at the Centers for Disease Control (CDC), also a controlling body in the syphilis study, convened a panel of medical experts to ascertain the continuity of the study. Of all the panelists, only one internal medicine professor expressed opposition, even though he was unfamiliar with the particular details of the experiments. Nevertheless, the professor was overruled by the commission and the study was allowed to continue (Lederer, 2005, p. 21). A short time later, in 1972, news of the USPHS Syphilis Study was released by the media, prompting the assembly of another panel of experts. This time, the study was stopped by the Department of Health, Education, and Welfare (Lederer, 2005, p. 21).

When the USPHS Syphilis Study was exposed by the media, other questionable research experiments were known. Among these studies was the Willowbrook State School Study, in which children afflicted with mental retardation were administered hepatitis. Another research program involved children at the Jewish

Chronic Disease Hospital in Brooklyn. At this facility, patients were given live cancer cells without their knowledge or understanding (Lederer, 2005, p. 21). The revelation of these shocking experiments led to the enactment of the National Research Act of 1974. The act established several important requirements for human research subjects. One requirement was that potential research subjects must give written, informed consent before participating in research. Also, the act established the creation of Institutional Review Boards, which evaluated the efficacy of the study and ensured protection of human subjects. In addition, the National Research Act led to the establishment of federal commissions that analyzed the ethical ramifications of research involving humans (Lederer, 2005, p. 21).

Healing the Wounds of the USPHS Syphilis Study

President Bill Clinton offered a formal presidential apology to the survivors and families of the syphilis study at a White House ceremony (Shakir, 2011a). The event occurred on May 16, 1997 (Fairchild and Bayer, 1999). In another symbolic gesture of remembrance, the name of the study was changed to the US Public Health Service Syphilis Study (Shakir, 2011a). Finally, President Clinton issued an executive order calling for the creation of the Tuskegee University National Center for Bioethics in Research and Health Care (Shakir, 2011a). Despite the apology and other gestures, much needs to be done to heal the community. This will be difficult to do because the study did not affect just the men who participated. According to Shakir (2011a), countless women and families were affected by the study. Many women did not speak about syphilis because of the stigma associated with the disease (Shakir, 2011a). That stigma was complicated by racist and sexist stereotypes during that time (Shakir, 2011a). As a result, there are emotional injuries that are as acute as the physical injuries that the study participants endured.

Healing strategies are important because they address the issues that haunt both the living and the dead. Healing can soothe the pain of past memories and offer hope for a new beginning. These steps may be symbolic, because no amount of money or apology is able to erase years of hurt and mistrust. An excellent example of a healing strategy in Tuskegee and Macon County is Dr. Muhjah Shakir's efforts to use quilts to convey a pictorial account of the USPHS Syphilis Study. The quilts are part of a greater initiative to utilize oral history to convey the feelings of women as a form of catharsis (Shakir, 2011a).

Shakir believes that oral histories provide insight into the lives of the female descendants of the USPHS Syphilis Study. Also, telling these stories will break down the secrecy that these women have kept regarding the study and would provide, in the words of Dr. Shakir, a "catalyst for healing" (Shakir, 2011a, p. 36). The actual quilts that Dr. Shakir oversaw in her Tuskegee Syphilis Study Quilting Project were an extension of oral traditions. According to Shakir, the quilt is an artwork that has been utilized for years among women in the South. It is a way for African-American women to face their collective traumatic experience (Shakir, 2011a).

The quilting project developed by Shakir offered a form of holistic healing, because the making of the quilts gives the local women a chance to share their pain and to find peace.

According to Shakir (2011a), each quilt was made of twenty squares, each measuring 16 by 16 inches (Shakir, 2011a). One interesting quilt is entitled, *Doctors of Deceit* (Shakir, 2011a). In this particular quilt, the makers expressed anger at doctors who seemed to believe they were gods (Shakir, 2011a). Another quilt, *The Guinea Pigs*, weaved by the same women, described the anger of her entire town being used as guinea pigs (Shakir, 2011a). A third quilt by the same person was entitled, *A Volcano Eruption*.

In it, lava represents anger, rage, and death, among other feelings (Shakir, 2011a).

Quilts were not the only form of healing among the family members of the USPHS Syphilis Study participants. Dr. Shakir interviewed two focus groups during the Annual Commemoration of the Presidential Apology at the Tuskegee University Kellogg Conference Center during 2009 and 2010 (Shakir, 2011a, p. 105). Many of the women offering their oral histories were from the mother's side of their families (Shakir, 2011a, p. 105). Oral histories are important to understanding the effects of the study on the descendants because they open a window into their daily lives and struggles. Shakir (2011a) collected a number of oral narratives from female descendants. One such narrative described the life of a fifty-nine-year old woman who was one of six children growing up in Notasulga, AL. She attended the Shiloh Rosenwald School. However, she attended school intermittently because her services were required for growing season. The woman also attended Shiloh Missionary Baptist Church in the same community (Shakir, 2011a, p. 105). After graduating from Tuskegee University, she worked at the school in the grants department. The woman later worked at Auburn University (Shakir, 2011a, p. 106).

The forty-nine-year old woman stated that her paternal and maternal grandfathers, as well as her uncle, were study participants. Her maternal grandmother died in her forties from hemorrhaging (Shakir, 2011a, p. 106). The woman then stated that she lived with her mother. In addition, her grandfather, who went blind, and his two mentally disabled sons moved into her home. Between her five siblings, two cousins, grandfather, and father, the woman grew up with ten people in her three-room house (Shakir, 2011a, p. 106). The woman's mother was described as a hard working farm laborer who looked after the entire family. Her father supplemented the family income by bootlegging liquor.

Through his illegal business, the woman was able to know some of the USPHS Syphilis Study participants (Shakir, 2011a, p. 106).

Shakir (2011a) then detailed some of the feelings that the woman felt about the USPHS Syphilis Study. When asked if the community felt ashamed about the study, the woman stated that they should not have to feel any stigma because they were not responsible for the study (Shakir, 2011a, p. 107). The woman also felt that because of the study, many African-Americans feel distrustful of clinical trials, even though there are IRB procedures in place. Furthermore, the woman believed that by the time her blind grandfather was finally compensated for being a study participant, he had dementia. Thus, the woman believed that the money came too late for her grandfather, and that his life was worth more than the compensation (Shakir, 2011a, p. 107).

Healing Through Deliberative Dialogue

Founded by Dr. Muhjah Shakir, Tuskegee University professor of Allied Health, the Black Belt Deliberative Dialogue Group promotes meaningful discussion among members of the local and surrounding Macon County, Tuskegee, Alabama, community. The Black Belt Deliberative Dialogue Group is a community-campus partnership sponsored by the Davis Matthews Center for Civic Life, consisting of Tuskegee University student interns, faculty, and members of the local community. Deliberative dialogues are action based, community oriented, democratic, and focused on discussing and proactively engaging problems in the community where input and action is paramount. Additionally, the dialogues build a capacity for thinking and acting on important issues that are of past, present, or future interest in the collective life of the community (Shakir, 2011b).

Since 2011, a series of deliberative dialogues have explored the lingering effect of the USPHS Syphilis Study on the Tuskegee/ Macon County community and beyond. Since the abrupt conclusion of the study in 1972, unanswered questions have persisted and unresolved feelings have remained among family members of participants in the study and the local community members. In a series of ten forums (2011–2012), the deliberative dialogue group provides the community an opportunity to heal, explore, and taken proactive actions toward significant past and present themes related to the syphilis study. The aim of the deliberative dialogues is "to make meaning out of this traumatic experience, to contemplate important lessons, and to provide the catalyst for reconciliation and healing" (Shakir, 2011b, p. 3).

On December 4, 2011, I, Obiora N. Anekwe, attended the initial deliberative dialogue session as a faculty member of the Black Belt Deliberative Dialogue Group. One family member of a syphilis study participant attended the program session.

Marking the initiation of the deliberative dialogue series, the program began with a ceremony giving respect to the African ancestors through (water) libations (Photograph 2), which symbolized the confirmation of healing through the ancestors. Within West African culture, water traditionally represents the healing of a community's collective mind, body, and soul in order to progress to greater enlightenment. Additionally, libations are known as a traditional West African sacred ceremony performed at important events in order to honor and remember the ancestors. After water is poured, the audience's collective response is "Ashé," which means "and so it is."

Guidelines were provided by Tuskegee University student leaders about the program, which consisted of an overview of the meaning of deliberative dialogue, group agreements, an expanded historical context of the problem, and a call to action. The film, *Deadly Deception*, which is about the impact of the USPHS Syphilis Study at Tuskegee was viewed by the audience with feedback and dialogue provided at various intervals of the film's progression. After viewing the film, the session leader, Dr. Shakir, provided the summation and led the evaluation of the film and how it could impact upon healing the community from the impact of the USPHS Syphilis Study.

At the session's conclusion, each audience member was provided a reflection feedback form that asked significant questions about how the film, *Deadly Deception*, was used as a learning tool for healing and reconciliation. During the verbal feedback session, most of the audience members agreed that such a film should be viewed by a wider audience, such as local elementary, middle, and high schools to inform younger people of the importance of the syphilis study and its ramifications. Additionally, it was agreed upon by the audience that more young people need to be aware and educated about the study's impact, because many local youth may have had family members who were actual participants in the syphilis study. Such awareness would educate young people about their local history, which eventually impacted the national landscape of bioethics.

Seeking More Than an Apology:
An Example of Healing and Reconciliation

During the early to mid-1900s, at least thirty-two states passed eugenics sterilization laws that allowed sterilizations based on sickness, epilepsy, or feeblemindedness (Armstrong, 2012). Today, only seven states have apologized to victims of sterilization. North Carolina sanctioned a eugenics program that sterilized more than 7,600 people between 1929 and 1974, which became the longest held sterilization program in the nation (Armstrong, 2012).

One African-American woman affected by sterilization in North Carolina was Ms. Lela Mae Dunston, who at the age of thirteen was sterilized immediately after she gave birth to her only child. The mother signed the consent form for sterilization because, like so many other women, she was told by a state social worker that if she did not sign for her daughter, her welfare benefits would be eliminated. The effects of her sterilization have affected her emotionally and physically. As Ms. Dunston says, "They gutted us up like hogs, dogs, and cats. And we ain't healed. I just keep praying, asking God to give me strength" (Armstrong, 2012, p. 76). Her words are indicative of a lack of informed consent and an infringement on the autonomy of women to make health decisions involving their own bodies frequently found in the history of such programs. Ms. Dunston's summation says it best: "They didn't have no right taking people's dignity and pride away" (Armstrong, 2012, p. 76).

Initially, most of the women who were sterilized felt powerless against the State of North Carolina's unethical medical practices, but some women, such as Ms. Nial Ramirez in 1973, filed lawsuits against the North Carolina Eugenics Board. She says that although her suit was not successful, the doctor who performed the surgery gave her a personal check for seven thousand dollars. Her fight for reconciliation was noticed by State Representative Larry Womble, who, since 2002, has worked with the state to secure monetary compensation to uninformed sterilization participants (Armstrong, 2012). "In 2010, Governor Bev Perdue established the North Carolina Justice for Sterilization Victims Foundation to help determine proper compensation for victims. Since then, seventy-two victims have been identified, but experts estimate that there are probably up to 2,000 still living" (Armstrong, 2012, p. 76).

Applicability to Research Administrators

The USPHS syphilis study is significant to research administration for three reasons. First, the plight of the family members of the former study participants is due to the negative effects of the study on them. Not only were the participants adversely affected by human experimentation, family members, such as participants' wives, contracted syphilis and were eventually stigmatized by the media attention that their community received when the study was exposed. Research administrators must understand how to address the material and social needs of participants and their family members affected by unethical research since they bore no responsibility for their misfortune. Second, by addressing the aforementioned needs, research administrators may be better able to deal with inevitable perceptions concerning the 1932–1972 syphilis study. Media coverage may have contributed to the current mistrust of the public health system by African-Americans. This mistrust is particularly disturbing because much current research that is intended to provide meaningful treatment for African-Americans is limited by low participation in clinical trials. Third, research administrators, acting on behalf of local health departments, can better coordinate research-related holistic healing strategies through rural and urban outreach programs designed to assist family members in seeking mental and physical treatment of diseases.

For many research administrators, the syphilis study also serves as an ethical and reflective learning apparatus in the medical, health-care, and related fields of study. Outcomes of the study affected the development of ethical concepts such as informed consent and the establishment of the Institutional Review Board (IRB) in modern research institutions and programs. If it were not for the original study's exposure and revelation in 1972, many laws protecting research subjects would not have been formulated and established to prevent future unethical violations in research. It is paramount that all emerging and seasoned institutional research leaders are aware of the positive and negative effects they have on research participants and their family members' holistic health and well-being. Only then, can all parties become more effective as leaders in the diverse fields of medical and health-care research.

Conclusion

The USPHS Syphilis Study in Tuskegee damaged the trust of African-Americans, especially African-American males, regarding public-health awareness and studies conducted by public health entities. In essence, the syphilis study reinforced distrust of the medical establishment and public health programs, and reinforced fear of vaccinations. As a significant result, many African-American families associated with the study still distrust the public-health community in general, and are, therefore, hesitant to receive preventive care or participate in future medical trials by public health officials and institutions.

As the development of comprehensive healing initiatives is solidified, it is hoped that holistic healing ideals will act as a comforter for families affected by the USPHS Syphilis Study, while honoring the sacrifices of their ancestors. Truth telling about the past and about the hopes for the future is central to these holistic healing ideas. Medical and health-care clinicians must understand, hear, acknowledge, and act toward on the needs of families affected by the USPHS syphilis study. Only then will holistic healing finally occur among those who have suffered so much due to unethical practices espoused by public health officials.

References

Armstrong, L. (2012, April). "Sterilized by the state," *Essence Magazine, 42* (12), pg. 74–78.

Berg, J. W.; Appelbaum, P. S.; Parker, L. S.; and Lidz, C. W. (2001). *Informed consent: Legal theory and clinical practice.* Oxford University Press.

Centers for Disease Control and Prevention. (2011). "Research implications: How Tuskegee changed research practices." Retrieved from http://www.cdc.gov/tuskegee/after.htm

Cook, B. and Jackson, T. (2012). "Eighty years of "bad blood": The evolution of human research after the Tuskegee Study." *Journal of Healthcare, Science and the Humanities,* 2 (1), 31–58. Retrieved from http://nmvaa.org/mhrl/sub-Page.php?sp=13

Fairchild, A. and Bayer, R. (1999). "Uses and abuses of Tuskegee," *Science New Series, 284,* 5416: 919–921. Retrieved from http://www.jstor.org/stable2899191

Javaheri, F. (2006). "Prayer healing: An experimental description of Iranian prayer healing," *Journal of Religion and Health, 45*(2). 171–182. Retrieved from http://www.jstor.org/stable27512920

Kirklin, D. (2007). "Autonomy and the role of metaphor," *Journal of Medical Ethics, 33*(1): 11–14. Retrieved from http://www.jstor.org/stable/27719774

Lederer, S. (2005). "Experimentation on Human Beings," *OAH Magazine of History, 19*(5): 20–22. Retrieved from http://www.jstor.org/stable/25161974

Marciano, C. (2001). "Holistic Ethics," *The American Journal of Nursing, 101*(1): 24A-24C. Retrieved from http://www.jstor.org/stable/3522284

Meyerstein, I. (2005). "Sustaining our spirits: Spiritual study/discussion groups for coping with medical Illness," *Journal of Religion and Health,* 44 (2), 207–225. Retrieved from http://www.jstor.org/stable/27512853

Notermans, C. (2007). "Loss and healing: A Marian pilgrimage in secular Dutch society," *Ethnology, 46*(3), 217–233. Retrieved from http://www.jstor.org/stable/20456626

Poloma, M. and Hoelter, L. (1998). "The 'Toronto healing': A holistic model of healing," *Journal for the scientific study of religion, 37*(2), 257–272. Retrieved from http://www.jstor.org/stable/1387526

Reverby, S. (2001). "More than fact and fiction: Cultural memory and the Tuskegee Syphilis Study," *The Hastings Center Report, 31,* (5), 22–28. Retrieved from http://www.jstor.org/stable/3527701

Riches, D. (2000). "The holistic person: Or, the ideology of egalitarianism," *Journal of the Royal Anthropological Institute,* 6 (2), 669–685. Retrieved from http://www.jstor.org/stable/2661036

Schoenbrun, D. (2006). "Conjuring the modern in Africa: Durability and rupture in public healing between the Great Lakes of Africa," *The American Historical Review, 111* (5), 1403–1439. Retrieved from http://www.jstor.org/stable/10.1086/ahr.111.5.1043

Shakir, M. (2011a). "Ancestral voices of the living, rise-up and claim your bird of passage: an oral history with Tuskegee-Macon County women descendants of the US public health service syphilis study," California Institute of Integral Studies, San Francisco, California, the United States of America (unpublished dissertation).

Shakir, M. (2011b). *Black Belt Deliberative Dialogue Series Booklet.*

Shavers, V. L, Lynch, C. F., and Burmeister, L. F. (2000). "Knowledge of the Tuskegee study and its impact on the willingness to participate in medical research studies," *Journal of the National Medical Association,* 92(12): 563–572. Retrieved from http://www.ncbi.nlm.nih.gov/pmc/articl es/PMC2568333/

Solomon, R. C. (2006, August). "Ethical issues in medical malpractice," *Emergency Medical Clinics North American Journal,* 24 (3), pg. 733–47.

Storck, M., Csordas, T., and Strauss, M. (2000). "Depressive Illness and Navajo Healing," *Medical Anthropology Quarterly, New Series,* 14(4), 571–597. Retrieved from http://www.jstor.org/stable/649721

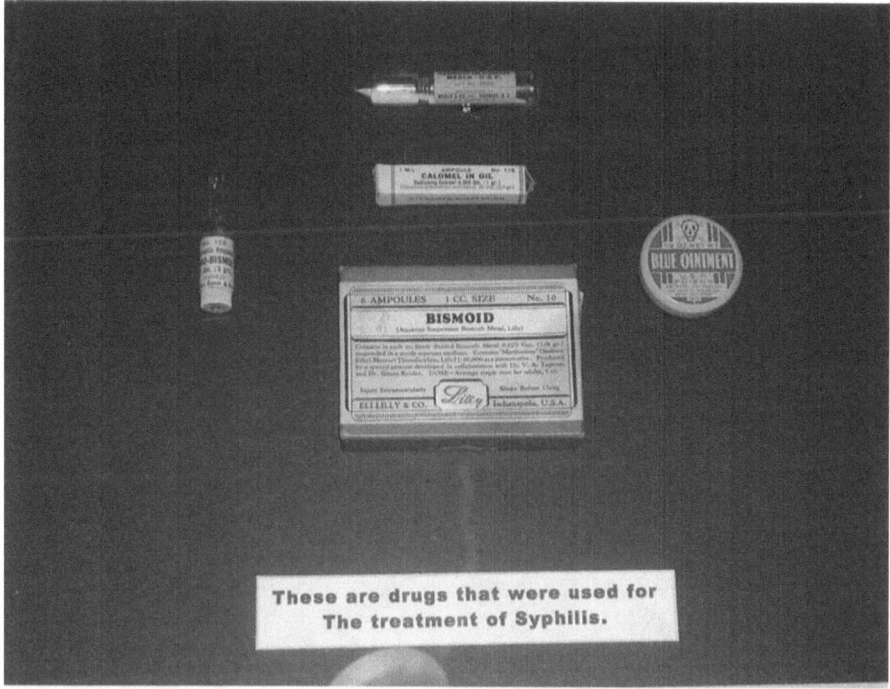

Photograph 1: *Display of drugs available for the treatment of syphilis, but were not used to treat patients with syphilis who participated in the USPHS Syphilis Study. Display Location: The Legacy Museum at Tuskegee University, Tuskegee, Alabama. Photographer: Obiora N. Anekwe*

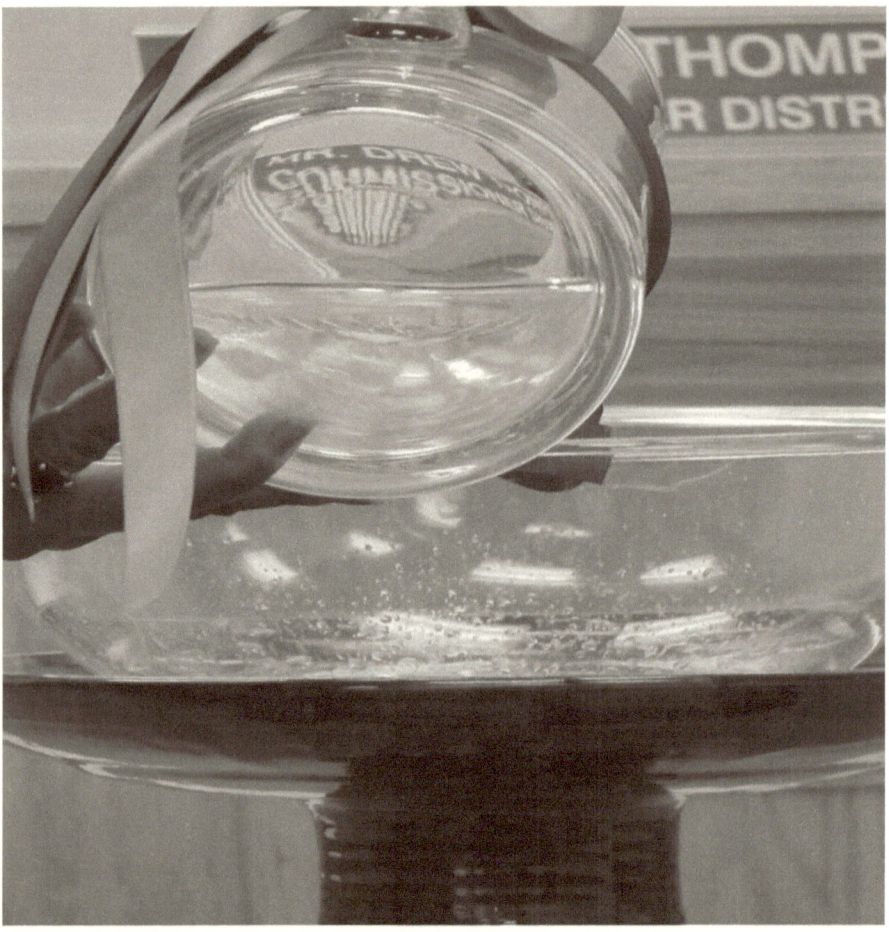

Photograph 2: *The presentation of spiritual libations of water, symbolic in African culture of healing. Presentation held on December 4, 2011 at a community dialogue in Tuskegee, Alabama, about the USPHS Syphilis Study. Photographer: Obiora N. Anekwe*

CHAPTER 5:
BIOETHICAL COMMENTARIES

What Should the Tuskegee Syphilis Study Be Called?

As I began to conduct research on the Tuskegee Syphilis Study a few years ago, there was some discussion about renaming it. The debate ignited when some critics did not want the syphilis study perpetually affiliated with the facility where the study was conducted. These critics argued that the usage of the word *Tuskegee* unfairly suggested that Tuskegee Institute (now Tuskegee University) was complicit in the sponsorship of the syphilis study. The study has been historically known by other names, such as the US Public Health Service Syphilis Study at Tuskegee, the Tuskegee Study of Untreated Syphilis in the Negro Male, and the Tuskegee Experiment.

All these names make reference to *Tuskegee* as the source location of the study itself. The clinical headquarters for the syphilis study was at the John A. Andrew Memorial Hospital on the campus of Tuskegee Institute in Alabama. The syphilis study was conducted from 1932 until 1972. The hospital was founded in order to treat the university and local community because of segregation laws that did not allow African-Americans to be treated at white only hospitals. In some cases, African-American patients could be treated in segregated wards in some hospitals in the Southeast.

There are several undisputed facts. The study was sponsored by the US Public Health Service Department, but in large measure, Tuskegee Institute agreed to the nature and content of the research agenda. In large part, there were a number of administrative and medical staff personnel who were paid by the federal government to assist in coordinating the efforts and goals of the study. One Tuskegee Institute employee, Eunice Rivers, was a nurse on loan from the school to assist in the recruitment of male participants and the everyday operation of the study. Without the approval of Tuskegee University, the study could not have been conducted. Without the usage of the hospital facility, the syphilis study would not have persisted and expanded throughout its forty-year tenure as a clinical trial.

If we eradicate the usage of the word *Tuskegee* from the syphilis study, we will deny the existence of its full story and nature. Therefore, we would be unethical in our own depiction of history and further dishonor the lives of the African-American men who were victims of study if we were to remove the word *Tuskegee* from it. I argue that we must embrace our full history, which tells a story that we sometimes do not want to embrace. In order to properly heal from the wrongdoings of the past, the word *Tuskegee* should be maintained in order to preserve the authenticity of medical history. I also argue that if we exclude the word *Tuskegee* from the title of the syphilis study we would dislocate the study and fail to provide a geographical reference point for people who are unfamiliar with the study's background. In essence, to drop the word *Tuskegee* from the name of the syphilis study would be to rewrite history, which is unethical and biased.

In order to progress and provide healing to family members of the victims of the syphilis study, we have to face the atrocities of the past and move forward toward the future. As an old proverb states: we must know our past in order to know our future. Our past is *our* past, with its good and bad features. It affirms that we have a history that cannot be taken away. We must remember the ancestors who literally sacrificed their lives, even when they were not aware of the full extent of their medical sacrifice.

~ Obiora N. Anekwe

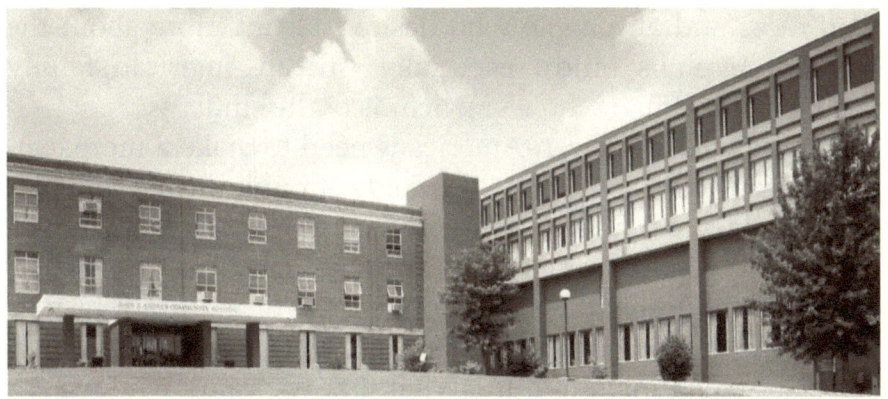

Photograph of John A. Andrew Memorial Hospital. Source: Tuskegee University Archives, Tuskegee, Alabama

Should White Scholars Write about the Tuskegee Syphilis Study?

In recent years, the historical findings, research investigations, and additional bodies of work related to the Tuskegee Syphilis Study have been produced primarily by white American scholars. By default, a white face has been put on the scholarship of an unethical study that affected black men with syphilis. The Tuskegee Syphilis Study was conducted mostly by white health-care officials. Such an irony is likely to promote an unintentional research bias and the possibility of a one-dimensional interpretation of the Tuskegee Syphilis Study. There is no question that white scholars should be able to conduct research on the Tuskegee Syphilis Study, but the larger question is do they have the right to dominate the re-search agenda?

I contend that racial diversity among scholars who research the syphilis study is so lacking that the mentoring of trained African-American scholars is needed in order to promote a more balanced perspective on the agenda of research into the study. The diversity of researchers who explore and write about the Tuskegee Syphilis Study should also be more inclusive of women of all races and all people who desire to learn more about the Tuskegee Syphilis Study, especially African-American family members of the men who were victims of the study.

In my opinion African-Americans need to make a more con-scious effort to do research in the fields of public health and bio-ethics in order to train a new, emerging group of scholars who are prepared to conduct research on the syphilis study. In essence, we need to educate ourselves about our own significant history rather than allowing other people to tell our story, no matter their race or research intention. It is vital that we value who we are and what our contributions were and continue to be in all sci-entific endeavors. It is incumbent upon us that older and more experienced African-American scholars mentor and share their knowledge about the Tuskegee Syphilis Study in order to further interpret the oral and written traditions dealing with the study.

Whether intentional or not, a Eurocentric interpretation of the Tuskegee Syphilis Study gives an inaccurate perspective to younger African-Americans who may want to conduct research on the study. If young African-American students are not taught properly about the syphilis study from a more balanced research perspective, they may unconsciously believe that only white-ness brings validity to research about their own culture. In other words, mental slavery is further consciously and unconsciously perpetuated upon younger African-Americans, which sends a si-lent but deliberate message that their voices are not welcomed or critically sought after. To date, I am not aware of any community in which the race that committed medical crimes upon a group of people dominates the discussion of its research agenda.

As we all are aware, knowledge is the greatest weapon for change. White researchers should join us in telling the story and spreading knowledge about the Tuskegee Syphilis Study, but their voices should not be in the majority. In order to effectively interpret the research agenda concerning the Tuskegee Syphilis Study, African-American scholars and researchers should be included in telling the story of how the nontreatment of syphilis promoted a greater medical mistrust from the African-American community for public health entities and an eventual lack of participation in clinical trials. But more significantly, we all have the responsibility to tell the story of the ancestors who literally sacrificed their lives in order to participate in one of America's most unethical clinical trials ever performed.

~ Obiora N. Anekwe

Ms. Elizabeth Sims: The Impetus for Why I Research the Tuskegee Syphilis Study

It all began with a phone call. My mother, Emma Jeanette, called me one day to tell me about an article she read in the *Tuskegee News* about the work Ms. Elizabeth Sims was doing with her foundation, the Shiloh Community Restoration Foundation. Through some research, I contacted Ms. Sims to ask if I could meet her and talk to her about my own interest in the Tuskegee Syphilis Study. So I called Ms. Sims to request a meeting with her. She agreed, and we decided to meet at the Kellogg Conference Center on the campus of Tuskegee University. There she asked me quite a few questions, attempting to figure out my own family connection to Tuskegee, the college and the town. I told her who my father and mother were and how they once both worked for

Tuskegee University in the 1960s. As I talked, she remembered my father, in particular, because of her work in the grants office at the university. She stated that she would often help him through the process needed to obtain the research grants he wrote during his tenure as an associate professor in chemistry. Eventually she began to develop a sense of trust, because she realized that I had a personal family connection to Tuskegee.

One point I had to make with Ms. Sims was that my work was not connected to my status as a faculty member at Tuskegee University but rather to my graduate coursework in bioethics at Union Graduate College-Mount Sinai School of Medicine. This distinction was very important to her. She and other family members of syphilis study victims felt hesitant to work with Tuskegee University because of a complex relationship between the town of Tuskegee and its respective university. As Ms. Sims explained to me, many families felt that the university benefited both financially and materially from the nationally televised apology for the federal government's sponsorship of the Tuskegee Syphilis Study. Many family members of the victims also believe that the university's participation had never been reconciled and explained to them, which had created further tension between the town and the university.

During the time in which Ms. Sims and I interacted, she confided to me that she had cancer, but she was in a state of remission. There was a lot of work she was attempting to do in order to sustain her foundation. But nevertheless, she made time out to help me develop my initial project, which was to research the burial site at the Shiloh Missionary Baptist Church in Notasulga, Alabama, in order to determine if some men who were involved in the syphilis study were not formally recognized. She often told me that there were a few men that she personally was aware of who were not listed on the Centers for Disease Control and Prevention's listing of syphilis study survivors for one reason or another. I found this quite fascinating and desired to know more about this particular issue. At one point during a tour Ms. Sims gave me of the Shiloh Cemetery site, she pointed out several graves of these men and told me she believed research on these men was important and that it had never been done.

From that point, I began to develop a research agenda centered around the gravesites of the men who may not have been formally recognized for their participation in the Tuskegee Syphilis Study. I also began to integrate the theme of holistic healing as a means of reconciliation for the men and the other participants who are now deceased as well. Because many family members of these men told me personally that they did not feel that healing had completely taken place within their families, I also was determined to bring greater recognition to these families through an active set of healing initiatives, which would be developed over time.

The more I wrote about the Tuskegee Syphilis Study, the more driven I became to bring all my healing initiatives to reality. But in order to do so, I had to clearly explain to family members I talked to and formed relationships with that I only had sincere interests in the study. It took a great deal of perseverance and persistent to continue on this path of acknowledging the struggle these men and their families endured due to unethical medical practices of health-care professionals.

Ms. Sims and I became so close that she tried effortlessly to use her own personal connections in the local Tuskegee community to help me with my research project. She informed me of one local funeral home that had the records of some of the men who possibly were in the syphilis study but were never recognized. This would have been a major breakthrough in my research, but unfortunately, Ms. Sims died as a result of a long battle with cancer before we could further explore the topic.

I remember as if it were yesterday when I last saw Ms. Sims. On a weekday, I went to meet her at her home in Tuskegee to return some documents to her. She looked very tired. A week or two later, after being informed of her death, I realized that her cancer had come back and she was actually fighting for her dear life. Ironically, I received a personal note from her in my PO Box. It was a note of appreciation that I archived with my research documents in order to remember why I am working so hard to help tell the story of the syphilis study survivors and their families.

~ Obiora N. Anekwe

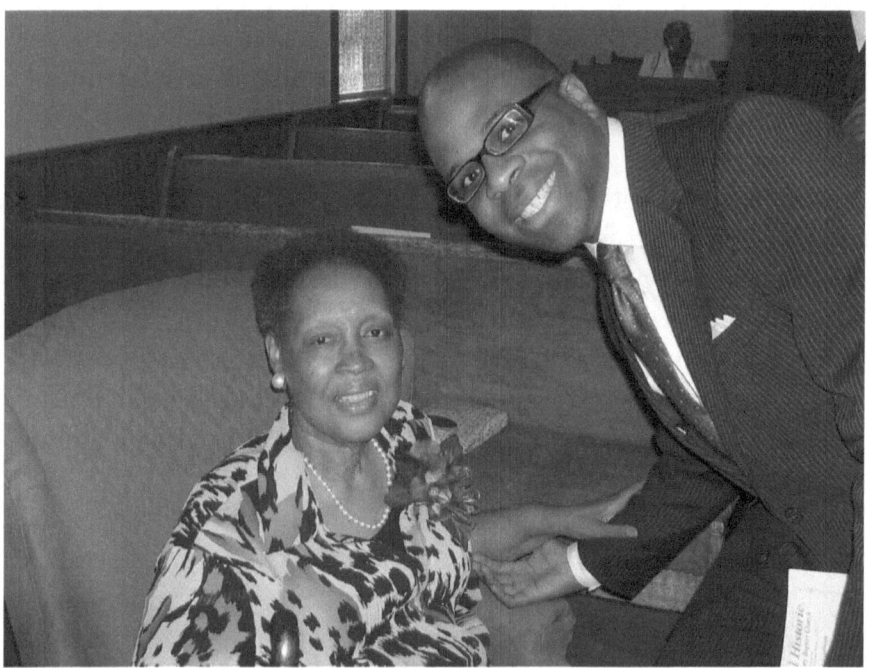

Photograph with Ms. Sims at a program celebration of her life. Location: Shiloh Missionary Baptist Church

Causing Medical Harm, Doing Medical Good

Is it possible to cause medical harm to one segment of a popu-lation, while creating medical good for another? In the medical cases involving the Tuskegee Syphilis Study and the treatment of children with polio, this point is quite evident. History itself has proven that it is possible for medical healers to cause the greatest harm to one group of patients, while systematically providing the greatest medical good to another. Two medical incidents are examples of such a dichotomy at the John A. Andrew Memorial Hospital at Tuskegee Institute (now Tuskegee University) in Alabama.

Originally established in 1892, the hospital (formally known as the Tuskegee Institute Hospital and Nurse Training School) was founded as Alabama's first hospital for African-Americans. It served the university community and trained black nurses during a period in American history when local hospitals were racially segregated or just plain did not serve African-American patients. When Dr. John A. Kenney was appointed in 1902 to serve as the hospital's director, its role expanded and it began to serve the surrounding local community as well.

Interestingly enough, during the same time the syphilis study took place, the hospital itself treated children who had polio. Many medical facilities in the South did not treat black children with polio because of racial segregation during the height of the polio epidemic in the 1940s and 1950s. Therefore, the John A. Andrew Memorial Hospital became the main medical facility in the Southeast that treated these children. Handmade walking braces and the warm waters of the hospital's swimming pool provided young patients with the care they needed to cope with symptoms associated with polio. The crutches physically helped children who were treated for polio in the Infantile Paralysis Unit of John A. Andrew Memorial Hospital. But unfortunately, while these young children were being cared for, patients with syphilis suffered under the care of some medical officials who refused to provide medical care for them. The hospital staff conducted medical good, but there was a segment of the medical population at the hospital who also participated in the nontreatment of black men. Nonetheless, the two main forms of medical practice that occurred in the John A. Andrew Memorial Hospital were medical harm and medical good.

As we can see so far, whether intentional or not, we can do more harm than good. As previously discussed, in the case of the Tuskegee Syphilis Study, medical professionals withheld medical treatment from patients with syphilis throughout a forty-year period. Often times, we may hear about these mistreatments, but at times, we need to divinely know about such stark examples of the effects of nonmedical treatment in order to make a difference for all people who suffer.

~ Obiora N. Anekwe

Tuskegee Remembered: The Collective Memory of Our Ancestors

In all we do and all that we are, we carry the memory of our ancestors with us. Even in our most sacred and intimate spaces, they are alive. There can be no denial that our ancestors lived and, to some extent, haunt us. Central to this truism, I reflect upon the written works of Rabbi Abraham Joshua Heschel and Chinua Achebe in the literary works *Israel: An Echo of Eternity* and *Things Fall Apart*, respectively. These works of prose are distinctly different, but their overarching theme deals with remembrance and how memory for one's own people and native land is connected to human memory and existence.

No matter where we are or who we become, home is where the heart is and home is where we meet the sacred nature of God. The Jewish and Igbo people are inextricably linked because of their historical search for statehood. Known as the Jews of Africa, the Igbo people have struggled to survive and to thrive collectively, both economically and educationally.

Indifference and inhuman injustice have displaced African-American people in America as well, especially African-American men, who have become an almost extinct population. The prison-industrial complex, addiction to illegal drugs, and internalized criminal violence have become the mental and physical chains that have stifled the capacity of many African-American men who seem to be left in a world without hope. The collective memory of our ancestors speaks to and through us and tells us that we are not bound by our human existence, but rather we all have the human capacity to overcome unbearable odds.

One of the most disturbing facets of the Tuskegee Syphilis Study is not its medical implications, which are significant, but its psychological impact on the African-American male population. These men who were involved in the study experienced a spiritual holocaust and psychological colonialism that affected generations upon generations of African-American males. These men became a representation of how systematic evil, void of justice, can destroy a segmented population through human myth and systematic racial prejudice. Medicine was simply a tool to carry out these evils.

Remembrance, though, brings forth the ability to begin healing from the past, but only if remembrance is righteous. In order to remember the Tuskegee Syphilis Study respectfully, one has to be cognizant of the spiritual nature of the African-American community and the nature of the African-American male within that community. Most of the African-American men who participated in the study were recruited from the most sacred place within black culture: the black church. Many of these same men were also buried in cemeteries that were near or at their churches. Therefore, the voices of these ancestors still speak from the grave.

I believe that their voices are unsettled and yearn for the healing of their descendants who still suffer and seek healing themselves. Most pained are the unheard and ignored voices of their sons, who have internalized the disrespect of the sacred nature of trust and exchanged it for despair and hopelessness. Just as the Igbo soul sought for a home, just as the Jew sought for refuge in his homeland, so does the African-American male seek the comfort of his male ancestors from the human atrocities of this world.

~ Obiora N. Anekwe

Building Trust in Public Health Ethics

In my readings of a recent article by Blendon et al (2006), I was intrigued by the point the authors made about the fact that African-Americans who were surveyed stated that they were less likely to trust government officials, in particular, public-health officials. The authors highlighted that their lack of trust may be rooted in discriminatory actions taken by public-health officials in the past. When I read these statistics, I immediately thought about the Tuskegee Syphilis Study and how it significantly affected the way in which African-Americans view public-health officials. In reality, African-Americans' mistrust of public-health officials is quite appropriate and is still evident today. Public health officials continue to struggle to develop strategies in order to increase the number of African-Americans who participate in public-health studies.

One suggestion Blendon et al recommended in order to increase the number of African-American participants in clinical trials is to increase the role of African-American public-health officials in recruitment efforts. Although their suggestion may be noble, it is historically misguided. As the Tuskegee Syphilis Study demonstrated, African-American public-health officials were also involved in unethical clinical trials, such as Nurse Eunice Rivers and other African-American officials who worked for and with the US Public Health Service during the height of the Tuskegee Syphilis Study. Even today, mistrust by the African-American community continues to exist because many African-Americans feel betrayed by African-American public-health officials who also played a significant role in the Tuskegee Syphilis Study.

Blendon et al's argument could be enhanced if they recommended that trust may be rebuilt within the heart of the African-American community through the black church, which was the main recruitment ground for the men who participated in the Tuskegee Syphilis Study, and which continues to serve as the bedrock of trust within the black community. If public health officials begin within the black church, I believe that trust within the black community may be rebuilt in order for more African-Americans to participate in public health studies again.

~ Obiora N. Anekwe

Reference

Blendon, R. J., DesRoches, C. M., Cetron, M. S., Benson, J. M., Meinhardt, T., and Pollard, W. (2006). "Attitudes toward the use of quarantine in a public health emergency in four countries," *Health Affairs*, pgs. 15-25.

Upon My Return: Revisiting What Has Been Studied Before

In life, we seldom return back to where we began. But for researchers, especially anthropologists and ethnographers, revisiting and rediscovering past encounters seems to be commonplace. As researchers, we are trained to keep a healthy distance from our subjects. We are also trained to only think of our subjects as data or numbers that lead to the answers we seek. Anthropology tends to solicit a different kind of response. Rather, returning to what we once explored is not only common, but at times required in order to reexamine our contextual knowledge of the subject matter we so vividly explored. But in the article titled, "Revisits: An Outline of a Theory of Reflexive Ethnography," author Michael Burawoy describes a different type of revisit, one that entails revisiting a subject matter from a different researcher's perspective in order to frame a previous research dynamic in a different way and discover new and fresh insights.

As I have evolved as a researcher, I have begun to view my own research more and more as functional within a bioethical framework, while orientating myself through an anthropological scheme in order to seek my own unfound discoveries. Although there have been exhaustive amounts of research conducted on the Tuskegee Syphilis Study, there has never been one in which a trained bioethicist comes from an "insider's perspective" in order to interpret the knowledge we now know about Tuskegee. My background of being born at the very hospital in which the syphilis study took place provides a unique opportunity for me to frame research questions that have not been explored. Just as Michael Burawoy details in his own experience as a factory worker researching his topic, my concrete experiences as a child of Tuskegee and as a former faculty member at Tuskegee University allows me to see Tuskegee from both an insider's and outsider's perspective, now that I reside in Brooklyn, New York.

But as I have become more and more involved in my own research on the Tuskegee Syphilis Study, some may reasonably question how I distinguish myself as a researcher and viably contend with my own personal connection to the study itself? One way in which my personal role and that of researcher has been distinguished has been through my physical distance from the environment in which the syphilis study took place. I reside in New York City, a contrasting physical and social environment very dissimilar from Tuskegee. Therefore, my perspective has gradually evolved to that of "outsider" status rather than that of an "insider" mired in the environment in which I was born, attended graduate school, and worked as a professional for a number of years. Another factor to consider is my ethical education and training in the field of bioethics, which has built a substantial buffer against positive or negative biases that may influence research outcomes. This is not to say that we all do not have our biases in research, but it is to say that sound, ethical education in the field of bioethics has contributed to my development as a trained and observant researcher of issues related to the Tuskegee Syphilis Study. But more significantly, I believe that as a researcher my goal is to be a *truth teller*, regardless of my own personal or professional interests or stake in the project.

~ Obiora N. Anekwe

Reference
Burawoy, M. (2003). "Revisits: An Outline of a Theory of Reflexive Ethnography," *American Sociological Review.* 68 (5), pgs. 645–679.

Revisiting *HeLa*: A Family's Quest for Healing and Reconciliation

Earlier this year, scientists at the European Molecular Biology Laboratory published the genome of a line of HeLa cells, which made it possible for the public to digitally download the information through the Internet. The scientists made Henrietta Lacks's genome available to the public without consent from the family. Eventually, the researchers took down the public data from its website, but their actions call into question a need to reform privacy laws. But more significantly, the researchers' actions also shed light on the issue of informed consent for families such as the Lacks, who were unaware of the laboratory's unethical, but legal action of transmitting family genome data.

Henrietta Lacks was stricken with cervical cancer more than sixty years ago. Before her death in 1951, doctors who treated her at The Johns Hopkins Hospital in Baltimore, Maryland, extracted cells from her tumor without her consent. The doctors' cell acquisition procedures were considered legal at the time but in retrospect have been declared unethical. Recently, the National

Institutes Health (NIH) announced an agreement with the Lacks family that restricts NIH financed research on the genome of HeLa cells without the explicit consent of two family members on a committee that approves such research.

A significant ethical concern with the European Molecular Laboratory's Internet publication was the release of the full genomic sequence of HeLa that may reveal abnormalities in genes that could be transmitted to later generations. This brings into question whether it is ethical and even legal for families to own their full genome sequence. One disturbing, unresolved issue regarding the NIH agreement with the Lacks family is the fact that nonfunded NIH research entities can still publish the full genome sequence of the Lacks family without informed consent.

The policy efforts by the National Institutes of Health are progressive but, unfortunately, fail to address issues of healing and reconciliation for the Lacks family. Comprehensive informed consent policies need to be introduced in order to address contemporary privacy challenges such as Internet mass deliveries of family genome sequence data. But more directly, The Johns Hopkins Hospital, which treated Henrietta Lacks for cervical cancer and where doctors extracted her cells for research, should issue an institutional apology for their role in unethical research. To date, The Johns Hopkins Hospital has yet to issue such an apology, which in my opinion brings further shame to the institution itself and leaves the Lacks family devoid of holistic healing and future reconciliation. Although the NIH policy reform concerning family genome restrictions does not address all the ethical and reconciliation attributes of family healing, it is a start. At least now the Lacks family has a much deserved seat at the table of science.

A few years ago I had the opportunity of attending an exhibition about the HeLa experiment and the Tuskegee Syphilis Study at the Legacy Museum of Tuskegee University. At the time, I was a faculty member at Tuskegee University who also taught first-year students in orientation about the Tuskegee Syphilis Study. One of the correlations I taught my students was that both Henrietta Lacks and the men involved as research subjects in the syphilis study were from a social segment of working farmers who knew little about the nuances of science and medicine. They saw medical doctors as people who would help, not hurt them. So they trusted whatever their doctors said and did. It has been the premise that doctors involved in extracting Henrietta Lacks's cells and misleading the syphilis study participants believed that their medical actions were contributing to future scientific discoveries. But I have long held the belief that these doctors took advantage of people like Henrietta Lacks because they did not understand the physicians' true medical intents. Much of what occurred to these research subjects has more to do with health and educational disparities than anything else. It is shameful that in a health-care age in which Henrietta Lacks contributed so much to science and medicine so many of her family members still do not have basic health coverage.

Needless to say, the younger generation of Lacks have stepped up and reached within themselves to help educate others about their family saga. During the exhibition I mentioned earlier, I met Henrietta Lacks's grandson Ron. He spoke candidly and vividly about how his family, through the Lacks Family HeLa Foundation, has begun to tell the story about his grandmother—not to rewrite history but to heal as a family and prevent other families from being taken advantage of again. The foundation has become the vehicle and voice for his family to take a stand and help end health-care and education inequalities. I commend the Lacks family for their diligent efforts and truly believe that healing may finally begin to occur through their own acts of reconciliation.

~ Obiora N. Anekwe

CHAPTER 6

OTHER DOCUMENTED WORKS

A Proposed Lecture-Discussion to the Junior Scholars Program at the Schomburg Center for Research in Black Culture

The Ancestral Voices Series: Collages on the Tuskegee Syphilis Study and Beyond
Obiora N. Anekwe

From 1932 to 1972, the longest clinical trial in the history of North America took place in the small southern city of Tuskegee Institute, Alabama. Known as the Tuskegee Syphilis Study, it studied hundreds of African-American men over a forty-year period to measure the effects of syphilis in the black male body. Even after medications such as penicillin were discovered, these men were still denied treatment for syphilis. Many of them died from the effects of the disease. Today, all the African-American men who were study participants are deceased, but the family members of these men live on without their loved ones.

The goal of my proposed lecture-discussion is to tell the vivid story of these brave African-American men through the eyes of my art collages. The *Ancestral Voices Series: Collages on the Tuskegee Syphilis Study and Beyond* is proposed as a one-hour lecture and discussion that will tell the untold stories of the syphilis study through the unique perspective of the art collages I created through oral history interpretations, bioethical and public-health themes, and holistic healing initiatives for family members of victims affected by the Tuskegee Syphilis Study.

I propose to provide a thirty-minute lecture in a PowerPoint format that displays the various art collages I have created with explanatory summaries about each particular work. After the lecture, the students will have a twenty-minute interactive project activity that highlights the ethical and moral topics discussed during the lecture. Junior scholars will also have an opportunity to ask vital questions, during a ten-minute period, about the emerging field of bioethics, the Tuskegee Syphilis Study, and other pertinent topics that relate to the African Diaspora.

To date, there has never been a collage art series created that documents the Tuskegee Syphilis Study from an African-American perspective. This unique lecture presentation and interactive discussion with the junior scholars will provide a chance for students to consider bioethics as a field of study and provide a format for discussion and proactive actions on issues affecting black people globally. By this collective endeavor, the ancestral voices of the past can finally be heard and acted upon.

US Public Health Service Syphilis Study Survivors: An Ethical Analysis and Synthesis of Families in Healing
Obiora N. Anekwe

Research Overview
Goal: To create a national environment of healing through holistic initiatives

Objectives: The objectives of the study are:
- To identify syphilis study participants previously unidentified in the Centers for Disease Control and Prevention (CDC) list of US Public Health Service Syphilis Study participants
- To identify unmarked graves of these unidentified participants in order to place headstones on their graves
- To develop and create an educational mural on the Tuskegee University campus for the syphilis study survivors that creates greater awareness of what occurred as a result of the study
- To educate the public and grandchildren of syphilis study survivors about the legacy and truths of the US Public Health Service Syphilis Study

Outcomes: The outcomes of the study will be:
- To add syphilis study participants previously unidentified to the Centers for Disease Control and Prevention list of US Public Health Service Study participants
- To place headstones on the graves of previously unidentified syphilis study survivors
- To build an educational memorial on the Tuskegee University campus for the syphilis study survivors that creates greater awareness of what occurred as a result of the study
- To educate the public and grandchildren of syphilis study survivors in order to bring further awareness of the study to the next generation of young people

Methods: The methods used to actualize the stated objectives are the following:
- Library Research (conduct archival, government document research and define notions of *family* and philosophical ideals such as *trust*)

• Video (video taped interviews with additional syphilis study survivors, family, and extended family members to discover additional participants in the US Public Health Service Syphilis Study)

• Audio (audio taped interviews with additional syphilis study survivors, family, and extended family members to discover additional participants in the US Public Health Service Syphilis Study)

• Written Transcription (transcription of interview notes with additional syphilis study survivors, family, and extended family members to discover additional participants in the US Public Health Service Syphilis Study)

• Funeral Home and Cemetery Site Visits (visitation to funeral homes that house burial records and visitation to cemetery locations such as the Shiloh Cemetery in Notasulga, Alabama, to authenticate the burial and location of deceased syphilis study participants not listed on the original Centers for Disease Control listing of participants involved in the US Public Health Service Syphilis Study)

The objectives of the study will be realized in a three phases:

• Phase I (Year I): Data collection through library research, additional data gathering, and oral history interviews from key contact persons in the City of Tuskegee, Macon County, Alabama, and other parts of the country to determine the additional men directly involved in the syphilis study and the immediate/extended family members affected by the study. Critical to this phase of the research is to determine if the initial definition of family used by the Centers for Disease Control and Prevention appropriately defined such persons and family members.

• Phase II (Year II): Information gathered in Phase I will be analyzed and used to design appropriate interventions targeting the physical, social, psychological and spiritual needs of those families of the Survivors and their respective communities. For example, many of the graves of the men and some of their family members at the Shiloh Missionary Baptist Church cemetery have no headstones. Part of the healing ritual for family members will be to identify those graves and to place appropriate headstone on them.

• Phase III (Year III): Implementation strategies will be developed, implemented and evaluated to determine if a local healing environment has been created and what elements are generalizable.

The researcher will use a variety of research methods including but not limited to library research, video, audio, and/or written transcription of various data collected from various family members such as the wives and children of the Syphilis Study Survivors and plausible extended family members who were directly impacted by the study.

The ethical presupposition for this study is that the syphilis study participants' listing developed by the Centers for Disease Control and Prevention (CDC), which is routinely used to define and/or describe family, was generated for the purpose of extending medical benefits for "affected family members." However, the current list may exclude study participants who should be included, therefore increasing the number of known family members who may have also been affected by the syphilis study. The researcher will generate an additional listing with the names of additional family members such as the participants' wives, children, and additional participants who were impacted by the study. The nature and definition of family and extended family will be defined through a review of literature. Once the notion of family is thus defined, the researcher will be able to include additional participants and their respective family members in a working list of additional people affected by the syphilis study.

Significance and Impact of the Project

The Proposed Bioethics Research Masters Project is significant because it highlights the ethical obligations, or lack thereof, for moral and social justice in the fields of health care and bioethics.

The impact of the US Public Health Service Syphilis Study has had local and global implications in how research participants are informed during the research process.

But suspicion produced as a result of the US Public Health Service Syphilis Study is still evident in how community workers report mistrust of public health officials within the African-American community (Jones, 1981). The survivors and their families have been affected by the research negligence of medical practitioners who did not fulfill the medical mandate to first do no harm. Therefore, the goal of the research study is to provide a cultural environment of healing for additional study survivors and their families through holistic initiatives. The study will attempt to accomplish this goal by defining, through a review of literature, the notion of family / extended family, clarifying how a harm done to one member (such as through improper treatment) can have a significant effect on other members of the family, identifying the additional study survivors and their immediate/ extended family members affected by the study, recording the stories of the additional study survivors and their immediate/ extended family members, and identifying unmarked graves and placing head stones on them in order to begin the holistic process of healing from the results of the US Public Health Service Syphilis Study.

The study will produce several outcomes: 1) build a long standing relationship between the study survivors / family members, 2) identify unmarked graves of study survivors, 3) place headstone markers on the graves of study survivors, 4) identify the study survivors and their family members that were not previous known, and 5) build an educational memorial for syphilis study survivors that creates greater awareness of what occurred as a result of the study.

The research study will have an impact on how the study survivors view themselves and how their family members relate to the men involved in the study. In addition, the research study will have an impact on how the world views the role of the participants in the syphilis study. The identification of unmarked graves represents a sense of closure for both the study survivors and their families. In a sense, the buried syphilis study participants who are identified will finally be able to rest in peace and heal from the hurt and suffering the syphilis study produced. The greatest impact of the study will be in the children and grandchildren of the study survivors educating their own peers about their father/grandfathers' stories of survival. As future generations educate their peers, the myths that surround the syphilis study will hopefully be dispelled and stories will be shared through oral history interpretations.

Reference

Jones, J. (1981). *Bad Blood: The Tuskegee Syphilis Experiment: A tragedy of race and medicine.* NY: The Free Press.

Ancestral Voices: A Documentary
Obiora N. Anekwe
Fall 2012

From 1932 to 1972, the longest clinical trial in the history of North America took place in the small southern city of Tuskegee Institute, Alabama. Known as the Tuskegee Syphilis Study, it researched hundreds of African-American men over a forty-year period to measure the effects of syphilis in the black male body. Even after medications such as penicillin were discovered, these men were still denied treatment for syphilis. Many of the men died from the effects of the disease. Today, all the African-American men who were study participants are deceased, but their family members live on without their loved ones.

The goal of the documentary is to tell the vivid story of these brave African-American men through the eyes of their descendants. *Ancestral Voices: A Documentary of Stories from Families Affected by the Tuskegee Syphilis Study* is proposed as a one-hour documentary that will tell the stories of the syphilis study survivors through the unique perspective of the family members who knew them best. Several family members will be interviewed during a two-to-three-week period and asked about such things as why their loved ones participated in the study, what stories their relatives share with them about their experience in the study, and related issues.

The journey to document the voices and stories of families affected by the Tuskegee Syphilis Study began in 2010 with a video interview I conducted with Mrs. Elizabeth Ware Sims, founder and executive director of the Shiloh Restoration Foundation, Inc., and also a relative of many of the study participants. Her church community, the National Historic Shiloh Missionary Baptist Church in Notasulga, Alabama, was the recruitment site for many African-American men who participated in the Tuskegee Syphilis Study. Before her death in 2010, she gave me a tour of her church, the adjoining Shiloh-Rosenwald School, and the church cemetery, where many of the victims of the study are buried. The interview with Mrs. Sims and the tour she offered me provided me the initial idea to develop an oral history interpretation about victims and family members affected by the Tuskegee Syphilis Study. The following summer of 2011, I conducted preliminary telephone and e-mail discussions with some family members of the victims in order to target holistic healing initiatives that would assist in the psychological and spiritual healing of families affected by the Tuskegee Syphilis Study.

Family members have never been provided a platform to tell the untold stories of their loved ones who participated in the Tuskegee Syphilis Study. By providing a documented platform to voice their stories, the healing process for these family members will hopefully finally begin.

Letter to the Writer and News Editor of the *New York Daily News*
December 10, 2012, Unpublished,
in Response to Article Entitled, "Nazi Camp 'Art' Fury: Ghoul paints with victims' ashes"

Dear Mr. Siemaszko,

Yesterday, I read your article about artist Carl Michael von Hausswolff, who claimed that he stole the ashes of incinerated Nazi death camp victims. When I read this, I was very disturbed to say the least. As an artist myself who also traveled to the concentration camps at Auschwitz-Birkenau in Poland, I felt that Mr. von Hausswolff's actions were irresponsible, self-serving, and clearly unethical. I am an artist who believes that art can be used as an effective tool to provide a voice for the voiceless, but art is not a sanction for the degradation and devaluation of other human beings, especially those who have suffered under trying circumstances.

When I traveled to the concentration camps at Auschwitz-Birkenau, I was so greatly moved by what I saw that I began an art collage series about the Tuskegee Syphilis Study that went on for forty-years among African-American men who were observed, but untreated for syphilis until their deaths. This collage series also makes reference to the environmental similarities between the City of Tuskegee and that of Auschwitz, which made them both ideal areas to conduct crimes against humanity. These unethical research studies and evil acts cannot and should not be made a mockery of through art. Mr. von Hausswolff committed two terrible crimes. First, he stole the remains of another human being, and then he desecrated those remains. As artists, we are responsible for what our art produces, because it is a reflection of our innermost intimate opinions and beliefs about other people.

I commend you for sharing this pertinent story with the general public and hope this letter finds you well.

Sincerely,
Obiora N. Anekwe
graduate student in bioethics
Columbia University in the City of New York

US Public Health Service Syphilis Study Survivors: An Ethical Analysis and Synthesis of Family Healing
Obiora N. Anekwe
- Researcher born, 1974: John A. Andrew Memorial Hospital.
- Research Foundation: Applied Bioethics, Anthropological Studies and Oral History.

Goal
- To create a national environment of healing through holistic initiatives

Objectives
- To determine the criteria and to assess the acceptability of healing initiatives or strategies with family members
- To determine and compare the definition of family according to the Centers for Disease Control and Prevention (CDC) and the family members of study participants

• To determine the additional study participants who are not identified in the original Centers for Disease Control and Prevention (CDC) listing

Methods
• Library Research (conduct archival, government document research and define notions of family and philosophical ideals such as Trust)
• Video (video taped interviews with additional syphilis study survivors, family, and extended family members to discover additional participants in the US Public Health Service Syphilis Study)
• Audio (audio taped interviews with additional syphilis study survivors, family, and extended family members to discover additional participants in the US Public Health Service Syphilis Study)
• Written Transcription (transcription of interview notes with additional syphilis study survivors, family, and extended family members to discover additional participants in the US Public Health Service Syphilis Study)
• Funeral Home and Cemetery Site Visits (visitation to funeral homes that house burial records and visitation to cemetery locations such as the Shiloh Cemetery in Notasulga, Alabama, to authenticate the burial and location of deceased syphilis study participants not listed on the original Centers for Disease Control listing of participants involved in the US Public Health Service Syphilis Study)

Phases of the Study
• Phase I (Year I): Data collection through library research, additional data gathering, and oral history interviews from key contact persons

- Phase II (Year II): Information gathered in Phase I will be analyzed and used to design appropriate interventions targeting the physical, social, psychological and spiritual needs of those families of the survivors and their respective communities (ex. Identification of survivors' gravesites/placement of headstones)
- Phase III (Year III): Implementation strategies will be developed, implemented and evaluated to determine if a local healing environment has been created and what elements are generalizable

Community Outcomes
- To build a long-standing relationship among the living study survivors and their respective families
- To build an educational memorial for the syphilis study survivors that creates greater awareness of what occurred as a result of the study
- To educate the grandchildren of syphilis study survivors in order to bring further awareness of the study to the next generation of young people

Research Outcomes
- To identify the study survivors and their family members who were not previously known
- To identify unmarked graves of study survivors
- To place headstone markers on the graves of study survivors

Bioethical Outcomes
- To add syphilis study participants previously unidentified to the Centers for Disease Control and Prevention list of US Public Health Service Study participants

- To assist additionally identified syphilis study survivors and their family members in receiving reparations for participation in the US Public Health Service Study
- To provide holistic healing to additional syphilis study participants and their family members

Impact of the Study
- How the study survivors view themselves and how their family members relate to the men involved in the study
- How the world views the role of the participants in the syphilis study
- To what degree the children and grandchildren of the study survivors educate their own peers about their father/grandfathers' stories of survival

Review of Literature
- Definition of family and extended family members
- The placement of a permanent headstone for author Zora Neale Hurston (Fort Pierce, Florida, 1973)
- A Comparative analysis of resilience, self-identity, courage and the concept of invisible men involved in the syphilis study as relational to Jewish survivors of the Holocaust
- Exploration of the ethical concepts of *trust* and *mistrust* (ex. the oral history and anthropological studies explored in the Southern stories detailed in Alice Walker's *The Color Purple* and Zora Neale Hurston's *Their Eyes Were Watching God*)

Bioethical Assumptions
- Peter Singer, the Ira W. DeCamp Professor of Bioethics at Princeton University, would contend that the US Public Health Service Syphilis Study was unethical due to the pain

and suffering incurred by syphilis study participants without informed consent.

- The prevention of pain and suffering is a common theme infused in the applied bioethical framework of Professor Singer.
- The goal of medicine is to cure ills, prevent harm, and do no harm.
- The US Public Health Service Syphilis Study was unethical for a variety of reasons, most noticeably because the study promoted illness by not treating study participants, incurring harm to study participants, and encouraging harm to the syphilis study participants and the control group of participants.
- Healing is a primary benefit of health care and medical practice.
- The bioethics research project must be inclusive of the fields that are relational to health care, medicine, law, education, ethics, history, anthropology, and music in order to accurately transmit the outcomes of the project.
- Holistic healing is inclusive of the act of placing headstone markers on the grave sites of unknown syphilis study participants (what the researcher may refer to as "invisible men").
- The lack of headstones for syphilis study victims who participated in the study was a breach of contract between the participants and the US Public Health Service because a primary benefit of participation in the study was a guarantee of the proper burial and headstone after death.
- Proper death burial is a rite of passage and a completion of the cycle of life.
- The ethical implications of black male identity as identified within the Ralph Ellison novel, *Invisible Man* (1952), will solidify the assumption that black males were mentally

ignored in society, but physically used by the same society to promote the good of societal and medical progress through participation in the US Public Health Service Syphilis Study (1932–1972).

- *Invisible Man* was written by Ralph Ellison (1952) during the height of participation of black men in the syphilis study.

- The nontreatment of black males with syphilis in the study was as dehumanizing in practice as the lynching of black males in the South from the 1930s to the 1970s. Note: Tuskegee University has the largest depository of records relational to lynching during this period.

- The central concern of black male participation in the syphilis study and the lynching of black males is relational to the bioethical issue of death and dying. (Who chooses death? How does one die?)

Vassar College Black Cemetery Project

- Students in the African-American history class of Quincy T. Mills at Vassar College in Poughkeepsie, New York, teamed up with students of earth science and geography on a research project at the Negro Burial Ground in Rhinebeck, New York.

- The students used high-tech geophysical equipment at the half-acre cemetery and determined that there were far more people buried there than grave markers indicated.

- A simultaneous search of historical documents found that there was a vibrant black community in Rhinebeck in the nineteenth century, including a large colony of artisans.

Reference:

The Journal of Blacks in Higher Education (2010).

Truth Telling: Ancestral Voices of Families Affected by Clinical Research Conducted in the Tuskegee Syphilis Study

Obiora N. Anekwe

Abstract:

Medical researcher and virologist Jonas Salk once said, "Our greatest responsibility is to be good ancestors." His words reflect the belief that we are ethically responsible and universally connected to our communal families. Even in the face of human misdeeds, we can become our next generation's greatest oral teachers for positive change. Experiments such as the Tuskegee Syphilis Study can serve as a positive example of the need for truth telling, or informed consent, which can benefit and reinforce ethical measures to protect human subjects in clinical research. The Tuskegee Syphilis Study serves as a unique opportunity for family members of former study participants to provide additional ethical solutions in how to prevent future unethical clinical trials.

The researcher plans to provide an ethical perspective in how to interpret the ancestral voices of former syphilis study participants for positive change in order to create an environment of holistic healing for families affected by the study. An analysis of the doctor-patient relationship, truth telling, informed consent, patient rights, end-of-life care, and ethical implications of clinical coercion and deception will be provided. The doctor-patient relationship will be analyzed in regard to clinical coercion and deception held within the study with special attention on how such an unethical clinical relationship eventually jeopardized the spiritual, mental, and bodily healing of family members affected by the Tuskegee Syphilis Study.

The researcher will emphasize how effective truth-telling methods in the doctor-patient relationship can provide greater results in medical good instead of the medical harm that comes through deception and coercion. Examples of such effective practices that counteract the initial belief of public health officials that clinical deception was the most effective means of reaching the best medical results will be explored. The researcher plans to create a greater awareness of ethical medical practices by healthcare practitioners that creates an environment of healing rather than harm.

Background Summary:

The Tuskegee Syphilis Study occurred from 1932 to 1972 among African-American males in Macon County, Tuskegee, Alabama. Throughout the forty-year clinical trial, some men had syphilis (399), while other participants in the study did not have syphilis (201). The commonality between members of both study groups was that none of the participants were treated for the disease. Even after penicillin was discovered to treat syphilis, the drug was withheld from all study participants. Nevertheless, neither population was properly informed about the full extent and ramifications of participating in the study.

The researcher will focus on how family members of former syphilis study participants can assist in developing holistic healing initiatives that will assist in reversing the unethical medical actions by US public health officials who conducted the study. As a result, the paper will serve as a clinical analysis for the researcher's prospective capstone research project entitled, *US Public Health Service Syphilis Study Survivors: An Ethical Analysis and Synthesis of Families on Healing*. Ethical concepts, such as truth telling, informed consent, holistic healing, and clinical deception will be explored and defined to assist the reader in understanding the extent of the subject matter.

The researcher's initial interest in the Tuskegee Syphilis Study developed in 1997 as a graduate student at Tuskegee University, when former US President Bill Clinton formally apologized to former participants in the syphilis study for the United States government's sponsorship of it through the US Public Health Service. The researcher's interest in the study is also rooted in the fact that he was born on September 10, 1974 in the John A. Andrew Memorial Hospital on the campus of Tuskegee Institute (now Tuskegee University), where the Tuskegee Syphilis Study was conducted.

Conclusion:

Since 2010, the researcher's bioethical premise has been that family members of former syphilis study participants should provide holistic healing initiatives that will further enhance efforts to compensate for the ethical, clinical, and medical injustices that affect living family members and deceased syphilis study participants. The researcher's hypothesis is based on primary research in the form of personal conversations and interviews with family members who have expressed a necessity and willingness to provide recommendations for holistic reconciliation.

Based on the researcher's prospective bioethics capstone project, two objectives exist, which include 1) to explore the issues of medical harm and social trust for family members of syphilis study participants in order to build holistic initiatives of healing and 2) to formulate a set of holistic healing initiatives for family members of syphilis study participants by conducting interviews with these family members.

Although these two objectives are not directly explored within this clinical ethics paper, it is significant to mention them in order to gain a perspective for future reference.

As detailed in the poster presentation, the researcher will focus on three overriding themes within the clinical ethics paper: 1) the doctor-patient relationship, ancestral voices of family, 2) holistic healing of family, 3) and truth telling (informed consent).

The research outcomes for the clinical ethics paper provides a platform in which varying perspectives of the Tuskegee Syphilis Study will be explored, such as clinical coercion and deception, informed consent, and truth telling.

The researcher will emphasize how effective truth-telling methods in the doctor-patient relationship can provide greater results in medical good instead of medical harm through deception and coercion. Examples of such effective practices, which counters the initial beliefs of public health officials that clinical deception was the most effective means of reaching the best medical results in the syphilis study, will be explored. As a result, the researcher plans to create a greater awareness of ethical medical practices by health-care practitioners and an environment of healing rather than harm.

Bibliography:

CNN. (2008). "Did Tuskegee damage trust on clinical trials?" Retrieved from http://cnn.com/2008?HEALTH03/17.clinical.trials.ap.index.html

Coy, J. A. (1989). "Autonomy-based informed consent: Ethical implications for patient noncompliance," *Physical Therapy*, 69 (10), pg. 40–47.

Dunn, L. B.; Nowrangi, M. A.; Palmer, B. W.; Jeste, D. V.; and Sax, E. R. (2006, August). "Assessing decisional capacity for clinical research or treatment: A review of instruments," *The American Journal of Psychiatry*, 163(8), pg. 1323–1334.

Fisher, J. A. (2006). "Procedural Misconceptions and Informed Consent: Insights from Empirical Research on the Clinical Trials Industry," *Kennedy Institute of Ethics Journal*, 16(3), pg. 251–268.

Goleman, D. (2003). *Healing emotions: Conversations with the Dalai Lama on mindfulness, emotions, and health*. Boston and London: Shambbala Publications, Inc.

Jones, J. (1981). *Bad Blood: The Tuskegee Syphilis Experiment. A tragedy of race and medicine*. NY. The Free Press.

Muhjah, S. (2001). *Ancestral Voices of the living, rise-up and claim your bird of passage: An oral history with the Tuskegee-Macon county women descendants of the US public health services syphilis study*. San Francisco, California: The California Institute of Integral Studies.

Solomon, R. C. (August 2006.) "Ethical issues in medical malpractice," *Emergency Medical Clinics North American Journal*, 24(3). pg. 733–747.